Freezing People Is (Not) Easy

My Adventures in Cryonics

Bob Nelson with Kenneth Bly and
Sally Magaña, PhD

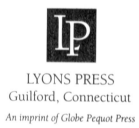

LYONS PRESS
Guilford, Connecticut

An imprint of Globe Pequot Press

Project editor: Meredith Dias
Layout: Maggie Peterson

Library of Congress Cataloging-in-Publication Data

Nelson, Robert F., 1936-
 Freezing people is (not) easy : my adventures in cryonics / Bob Nelson, with Kenneth Bly and Sally Magaña, PhD.
   pages cm
 ISBN 978-0-7627-9295-5
 1. Nelson, Robert F., 1936- 2. Cryonics. 3. Undertakers and undertaking—United States. I. Bly, Kenneth. II. Magaña, Sally. III. Title.
 RA624.N45 2014
 612'.014467—dc23

                          2013050225

Printed in the United States of America

10 9 8 7 6 5 4 3 2 1

This book is dedicated to Genevieve De La Poterie, a seven-year-old French Canadian child, beautiful beyond words. Genevieve was the world's first child frozen upon clinical death with the hope of future reanimation. In 1970 her Wilms tumor had no treatment and was usually fatal within three months. Today no child dies from a Wilms tumor, and it is completely curable. One week before her cryonic suspension, Genevieve, her mom, my daughter, and I went to Disneyland in Anaheim, California. On this occasion Genevieve spoke to me in French, through her mother's translation. She asked me, "Mr. Robert, would you please learn to speak French so I can explain to you directly why I didn't want to die so young and leave my beautiful family behind?"

This dedication also extends to Joseph Klockgether, owner of Rennaker Mortuary and the first California mortician to offer cryonics suspension services to his clientele. He's always believed that however a person chooses to be interred should be honored, be it cremation, burial at sea, or even placed into orbit like Gene Roddenberry, who is now circling our globe every ninety minutes.

This is simply every person's right of choice and must be honored by those entrusted to carry out this final act of interment.

Last, but far from least, are Sandra Stanley and Shelby Dzilsky. This couple allowed the frozen body of our first cryonics pioneer, Dr. James Bedford, to be stored in the garage of their Topanga Canyon home in dry ice for ten days while plans for his long-term encapsulation in liquid nitrogen could be arranged. Sandra also coauthored with Bob Nelson the book We Froze the First Man *and acted as his attorney during the appeal of one of the darkest times of his life.*

Sandra was a powerful force when introducing this new science of cryonics to humanity in the 1960s, the world and I especially owe her an enormous amount of gratitude for her contribution in the struggle to greatly extend the human life span.

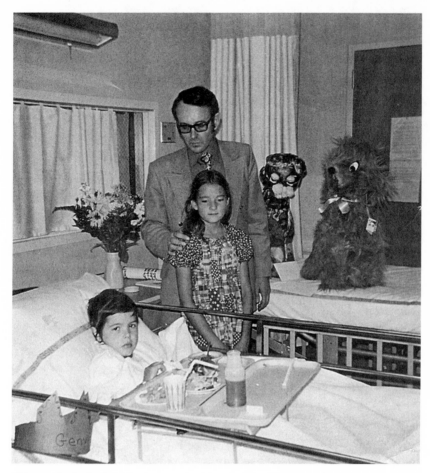

"Please, God, don't take me away from my family." The one and only time Genevieve spoke directly to me.

CONTENTS

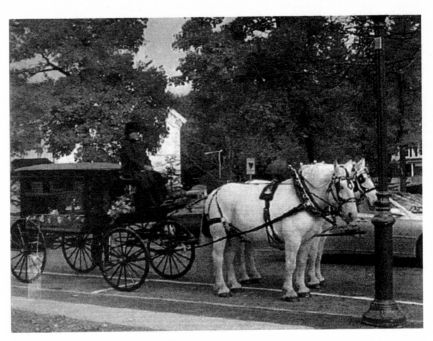

It calls for a change in perspective.

The Treasure Chest
by Kenneth Bly

Bob stood in the shadows of the garage, debating between fight and flight. I glimpsed the hurt and betrayal in his darkened eyes. He had locked away the memories in his mind with an even larger padlock than the one now sealing the crate.

He was anxious, looking away, his eyes distant and vacant. A lone lightbulb sent sharp shadows across the floor. Outside, an uncharacteristic Southern California rain pooled at the base of the wooden garage door.

The chest had remained sheltered in Bob Nelson's garage for twenty-five years. He had no desire to open it. Within its plywood walls, darkness shrouded the artifacts of a past life he had intended to shut away forever.

Moeurth, Bob's wife, rubbed his arm and said, "We don't have to do this."

I nodded but inwardly yearned to discover this hidden life. "Bob, we can do this another day."

"No," Bob replied, inching forward. "Too many years have passed. It's time to face my demons." He took the key from my waiting palm and bent down before the chest. He wiped a thick layer of dust from a section of the top lid, revealing the gnarled wood pattern beneath. A curious sort of magnetism permeated the air when he touched the crate. Like the telltale heart in Edgar Allan Poe's story, the contents of the treasure chest had their own story that needed to be told. Slowly, the key turned in the lock.

Bob was a pioneer; in the sixties he was the first to freeze a man and later several others, hoping they might one day be revived. He was one of cryonics' most prolific spokesmen until fate turned on him; he became reviled and retreated from his greatest passion for decades. I wondered what mementos from this past life could be inside the chest—certainly not a thawed body—but still I felt electric with curiosity.

Moeurth read my thoughts and spoke up, her sweet Cambodian accent soothing the tense atmosphere. "I had no idea either, Ken. We were married a year before Bob was able to tell me that he froze the first man, about his fame, and about how it all went bad."

For me the container was a treasure chest, but I could tell that for Bob it was something far more ominous. With the padlock discarded on the garage floor, he opened the lid, casting fresh light on long-obscured memories. The three of us leaned forward and peered into the crate. Looking back at us was a picture of a much younger Bob, shrouded in a cloud of dry-ice fog, newspaper articles, and the lead article in *Life* magazine. There were also audiotapes, reels of film, photos with Regis Philbin and Phil Donohue, and court documents from the cryonics trial—stack after stack of court documents.

Words jumped out at me from the newspaper clippings. *Pioneer. Swindler. Expert. Charlatan. Vanguard. Liar.* "Jesus Christ," I said.

Morosely, Bob replied, "I know."

"No, I mean that's what's written here from the court case: 'Bob Nelson pretended to be Jesus Christ with the power to raise the dead—all he needed was your money.'"

A flurry of thoughts tumbled through my mind as I delved into the depths of the treasure chest and into this mysterious and long-buried past. This wasn't just some embellished story that old-timers regurgitate at a bar; I was glimpsing the veneer of a complicated and painful odyssey. What an epic tale Bob had lived in those years!

I studied photo after photo in the treasure chest. Each fog-filled picture of his frozen heroes was permeated with the heady and optimistic belief that a doctor's pronouncement of clinical death was merely an interruption—not an ending. The cryogenic containers looked both crude and innovative, much like the old space capsules from the Mercury and Apollo programs.

That evening, I collapsed at home and pondered everything I had witnessed. I felt astonished again that, in our years working together, I never knew his true passions and heartache. It had always existed, buried deep by necessity but still inevitably influencing him every day since. I felt amazed that such extraordinary experiences could be locked in a dusty steamer trunk and stored for decades in a garage beneath boxes of old toys and unused kitchen appliances. We can never truly know what lurks in the hearts of people.

I had worked with Bob at his electronics repair center for seven years. He once mentioned that he had orchestrated the first cryonic suspension and written a book about the notoriety. I was dutifully impressed, but I wondered how he could have gone from scientific pioneer to TV repairman.

My mental image of cryonics was at once futuristic and sterile. I envisioned rows of stainless-steel tanks awash in bright, imitation light spilling from overhead fluorescents. Serious men with serious faces would mill about in white lab coats, busily fussing over the tanks. The people would be as interesting as the flat white paint adorning the walls of these subzero mausoleums. My exploration proved me wrong.

In the subsequent months, I spent hundreds of hours pawing through the contents of the treasure chest. I felt like a kid digging through my grandparents' attic. There was a letter from Peter Sellers, audiotapes of early cryonics conferences, boxes of court documents, and pictures and slides that were absolutely fascinating. I couldn't get enough!

I went online and searched for more about him, hoping I'd find more pictures and articles. What I found shocked and appalled me. I knew that Bob's organization had funding problems and that he was sued by family members of some of his frozen patients. In article after article he was described as a swindler. According to the stories, he had taken people's money and abandoned the vault where the bodies were stored, allowing them to rot. He had lied about his facilities and capabilities, claiming to have the world's first "cryotorium," but he had actually just dug a hole in the ground. He was given credit for freezing the first man, Dr. James Bedford, but that was all.

The mystery deepened. That description wasn't the Bob Nelson I knew. When I confronted him with the allegations one day in his living room, he only denied that he ran off with people's money. The rest was essentially true, but the intent was misrepresented, along with some of the details.

Bob was pensive. "For a quarter of a century, I've abandoned all my cryonics hopes. I was silent and allowed others to vilify me, fairly or not.

I haven't given my full account to correct history." Bob stopped, twisting an old newspaper. "For me, the Wright brothers' struggle to fly has a special poignancy. Most of their contemporaries rejected their experiments. The audacity of these mere bicycle mechanics, without even high school diplomas, thinking they could teach the world how to fly. I was a TV repairman; I wasn't a doctor or a scientist. Was it mere pride to consider myself qualified to freeze the first man?"

To answer that question, I went on a mission to find out everything, as much as possible anyway. I pored through court documents. I grilled Bob when I found inconsistencies in his story. His memory of the events was understandably less than perfect, and there were many holes to fill. To his credit, he was willing to accept information that conflicted with his recollections, and we were able to piece together a sincere accounting of what happened. I discovered such a fascinating, bizarre, and compelling story.

Bob Nelson didn't just coordinate the first cryonic suspension; he lit a fire under the cryonics movement. Although populated by intellectuals, scientists, cryobiologists, and doctors, it lacked a good front man. Cryonics was like the rock band Van Halen without David Lee Roth. Bob was slick, confident, and a little cocky. He was charismatic, and people naturally wanted to follow him. He brought an infectious enthusiasm for cryonics that bordered on lust. He was cryonics' first and, as far as I can tell, only rock star.

Bob's passion for cryonics and his drive to make it a success endured even when it was doomed. He just didn't know when to give up. After Dr. Bedford, there were more freezings, failures, and friends lost. His misguided actions led to a lawsuit that put not just him but all of cryonics on trial and gave the entire movement a black eye. Nevertheless, I hope that history eventually judges that what happened at Chatsworth was not a scandal but a tragedy.

CHAPTER 1

Growing Up Bob Nelson

I WAS BORN FATHERLESS IN 1936. During my childhood, my mom spent her time drinking, smoking Lucky Strike cigarettes one after another, or passed out from the previous night at her local bar hangout.

When I was five, my mom married a small-time Boston mobster, John "Fats" Buccelli. He was impeccably dressed, in specially tailored suits to handle his four-hundred-pound girth, and well-groomed, right down to the part in the middle of his hair. With his arrival and his subsequent departures to jail, my childhood fluctuated between the extremes of feast and famine.

John was tough and demanding, but he had one redeeming quality. He seemed to genuinely care about me, which is more than my mom could manage at the time. Early one morning when I was six years old, I heard a loud knock at the door. Three men with badges stood outside. John was under arrest for the armed robberies of several liquor stores. He was dubbed the "Lady in Red Bandit" for his choice of disguise while committing his crimes. But with his size, he wasn't hard to pick from a lineup.

The cops treated him well, perhaps because of his mob ties, and allowed him to make me some scrambled eggs before they took him away. John asked if he could write a note to my mom, who was passed out from a typical night of drinking, and he gave me a big hug before he was handcuffed. I was so sad that I couldn't eat those eggs.

I spent the next four years being shuffled from one dump to another and often left for weeks with strangers. Sometime after my little brother was born, Mom worked out a deal with her mom, Grandma Edith.

Grandma was a compact woman at five feet two inches and 150 pounds. Her hair was steel gray, and she had a heart to match. She was cheap too. Often she walked several miles into town to save ten cents on a loaf of two-day-old bread.

My baby brother, Little John, and I meant nothing more to her than the weekly twenty dollars she received to "care" for us. We spent the next two years forced to sit in a dirty, vomit-green overstuffed chair every day, all day; school wasn't a possibility. We couldn't even talk or go to the bathroom unless the witch gave us permission. Our only source of entertainment was to count the elevated trains that tore by the front window of the second-story apartment as we sat planted in our prison chair. On most days there were forty-seven trains from the morning until I was sent to bed at dusk.

One day the witch had been in a particularly bitchy mood, and Little John had pissed his pants because he was afraid to ask for permission to get off the chair. Grandma went into a rage and grabbed her wooden swatting spoon. She charged at John, swinging away.

I jumped out of my chair and got between them to shield him. My speed and audacity took her by surprise and threw her off balance. Her shock quickly turned to fiery wrath, and she reared back to strike me. Instead of putting my hands up in the defensive posture she had come to expect, I raised my little fists. My heart was beating frightfully fast, but I showed no fear.

I screamed at her, "Get away! Get away or I'll kill you, I swear!"

I was expecting at that moment for her spoon to collide with my head, but I had two years of pent-up energy and was prepared for battle. Instead she took several steps back and lowered her spoon-brandishing arm to her side. Her look softened a little as though she had expected a confrontation to happen someday. I was surprised, relieved, and emboldened at the same time. She said quietly, "Okay, Bobbie. I won't punish you or John anymore; I promise."

A week later she offered in a sweet tone to take John and me to play in Blackstone Park in the south end of Boston. In two years, she had never allowed us outside to play, let alone brought us anywhere other than to harass my mom at work.

The witch dropped Little John and me off at the Blackstone fountain pool. Regardless of her motive, I felt free. We laughed and splashed and chased each other. For a while we were just a couple of ordinary kids. When she returned at lunchtime, she set us on a park bench and told us to stay put until she came back.

We had become so accustomed to sitting in that damn vomity chair all day that we weren't concerned as the hours passed. When evening came, I realized she wasn't returning for us. I took Little John by the hand, and we walked for several miles in the cold to Grandma's small apartment. I held on tight to John, trying to ignore his chattering teeth.

When we arrived, I knocked on the door for a long time. We called for her, but the apartment remained silent and the door locked. Eventually the neighbor lady came out and said, "My goodness! What are you two boys doing here? Your grandma moved out today."

I knew it! I knew it! The old bag skipped out on us . . . hooray! With that information, I happily put my exhausted little brother on my shoulders and walked the three miles to my mom's work.

When I told Mom what Grandma had done, she sank down to the dirty bar floor, hugged us, and cried with shame. She left work early and took John and me home to her little one-room flat. It had a tiny kitchen, where she put a blanket down on the floor for John and me to sleep on.

About a month after we moved in with her, my mom told Little John and me that we had to go see someone who could help us. I made her promise it was not Grandma Witch, and she assured me it wasn't.

We took a long bus ride and arrived at a huge concrete office complex. Inside we met a well-dressed man. He took us into his office, which was small but neat. They discussed the abuse Little John and I had suffered while living with our grandmother. My mom told the man that she was sick, battling with the bottle, and had very little money. I was expecting this kind gentleman, who listened carefully to my mother, to give her some paperwork for government assistance. When he finally spoke, his response stunned and angered me.

"You can leave both of them with us. We'll take good care of them."

I felt betrayed. I spun around, looked at her in disbelief, and screamed, "You're giving us away, you bitch? You're giving us away? I hate you! I HATE you!"

I was upsetting her, but I didn't care. She wasn't supposed to send us away again. She rose from her chair, her telltale twitching indicating her need for liquid courage. I followed her to the door, hollering "I hate you!" as she raced through the lobby. I watched as she disappeared in the pedestrian traffic. Without so much as a good-bye hug, she was gone.

When I returned to the office, Little John was scrunched up in his chair crying. I felt terrible for him. I felt terrible for both of us. The man sat quietly at his desk and waited for me to stop crying.

Once I was calm and ready to listen, he explained in a soothing tone, "Your mother is incapable of properly caring for you right now. Bringing you to us was the best she could do. I've assigned you to a really nice lady who will find you a nice foster home." He stopped until he met my gaze. "I know it's difficult, but this is only temporary. As soon as your mother is back on her feet, you'll go back to her."

About an hour later an attractive lady came in and introduced herself as Miss Jane. She told us she was going to be our case worker and friend, and no one would hurt us again. We liked her and talked for hours.

That man had been nice. Miss Jane was nice. They were all nice, but it made me feel worse that my family was so nasty and neglectful. I held my little brother that entire night, battling feelings I was far too young to describe.

We drove around for the next four days, examined by one foster family after another. As I feared, no one wanted two boys. Miss Jane tried her best, turning down several opportunities for John and me separately. At the end of the third night, she told me we were running out of options, and she was probably going to have to backtrack and place us in separate homes, at least temporarily. I hated that prospect, but I understood. We had to accept that we couldn't be together.

On the fourth day we drove up to a large house in the middle of a small farm. We passed several cows, chicken cages, and countless rows of sprouting vegetables. A gray-haired woman came out to greet us. She looked just like Grandma Witch, and I felt a moment of panic, but this wasn't Grandma. She had kind eyes and was smiling, something I had never seen the witch do.

Miss Jane climbed out of the car and talked to the lady, Mrs. Brown, about Little John and me. I sat in the backseat and listened, squeezing my little brother's hand tight.

I liked this farm and this lady and didn't want any more disappointments, so I hatched a plan. As the two women approached the car, I whispered to John to hang on to me and not let go—no matter what. Miss Jane opened the door and saw John and I huddled together, clutching each other like Siamese twins facing the scalpel. Miss Jane tried to cajole me out of the car, but I wouldn't budge. Mrs. Brown opened the door on John's side of the car; they tried to physically separate us, but I braced myself against the seat, drew John closer, and held on tighter. We began to cry.

Frustrated, the women backed out of the car and regrouped. I heard Miss Jane apologizing for our behavior, sounding out of breath. They walked out of earshot and talked. After about ten minutes (which felt like an hour), they returned to the car. John and I steeled ourselves against another attempt to separate us, but Miss Jane only stood back and told us to come out . . . both of us.

John and I scooted out the opposite side of the car from where the ladies stood, still clutching each other, just in case this was a trick. Keeping her distance, Miss Jane explained that we could both stay, but only for a couple weeks. In the meantime we would have to work in the gardens and share a bed. There were fourteen other boys here; two of them would have to bunk together to make room.

John and I didn't hear anything past "You can both stay." We were too busy cheering, jumping, and running around in little circles. Several kids working in the garden stood up and watched the spectacle. We didn't care. We got to be together, and that was reason to celebrate!

Our two-week visit became a two-year stay. Mrs. Brown took a real liking to us. We worked hard at our many chores, but I didn't care after our two years of sitting. We played hard too. My favorite place was a huge pond on the property with fish, turtles, and frogs. I felt like Huck Finn on a great adventure. There was always something to do, something to be explored.

One day Mrs. Brown called Little John and me down to the foyer. Some barely perceptible hitch in her voice made me apprehensive— maybe it was the man from the foster agency taking us away, or worse, taking only one of us. I had long feared such a day would come. As I walked down the stairs, I saw a man spilling over the big couch in the living room, his back to us. He was a big man in a shiny pinstriped suit. When I recognized him, I jumped the rest of the stairs in a single leap, leaving my confused brother behind.

It was Big John, our dad! He hadn't forgotten us after all! I tore into the living room and dove into his arms. I was so overwhelmed; tears of joy ran down my face and dampened the soft fabric of his coat. He hugged me hard, and I inhaled his familiar aftershave. I could have stayed in this man's arms forever, but he eventually broke the embrace. I stayed close, not wanting to let go, but his attention was no longer focused on me. He sat perfectly still, staring forward. I followed his eyes and noticed Little John standing there, half hidden behind the wall. The two had locked eyes.

This was the first meeting between father and son. A big smile slowly formed on our dad's face. Little John just looked down at his worn shoes. Big John reached out, snatched his son into his arms, and held him for a long time. I felt a twinge of jealousy, but only for a moment. This man was, after all, his father too.

Within an hour, we were packed. I choked back some tears saying good-bye to Mrs. Brown. She had been so good to John and me, and we loved her for that. I gave her a big hug and ended that bittersweet chapter of my life.

John had rented a small cottage at a lakefront resort just outside Boston. When we arrived, our mom was waiting for us. She got down on her knees, swept Little John and me into her arms, and wept. Seeing her brought back cruel memories of all the times she gave us away, but I was still happy we were together as a family.

The initial bliss of our reunion didn't last long. Big John and Mom fought constantly about her drinking or his inability to earn an honest living. Within a year he got caught for bookmaking and loan-sharking and got his giant butt thrown back in jail.

I was twelve years old now and learning how to survive on the streets. This was a critical juncture in my life; I didn't want to go down the same path as my dad. Jail was not for me. We were broke, and often a twenty-five-cent package of bologna was dinner. I found ways to earn money and learned to be resourceful.

A group of neighborhood boys hung around a depot where big trucks offloaded fresh produce, and they would scoop up the fruit spillage for sale elsewhere. There wasn't any chance to move into this hustle—too many boys already. But I noticed several other truckers offloading at this depot, and most of them received little notice. The ones that caught my attention were the flower trucks. They spilled many perfectly good flowers that usually were swept up and tossed into large garbage bins.

I began surreptitiously picking up the flowers, trying not to attract attention. I didn't want my competition to copy my idea. Then I was off to the bars. I polished a quick spiel, pitching "Flowers! Buy a beautiful flower for your pretty girl!"

I was stunned at the instant success. This was fun, easy, and quite profitable. It provided real money that my mom and I used to eat and pay bills. Little John had been shipped off to family.

I was thirteen when Big John got out of jail and our family was reunited again. I was a different person than when he had left: a very seasoned young man, far from the typically sheltered American kid. Through hard work, I had taken care of myself and my mother. I was proud that I had succeeded as a kid where my parents had failed. While I had great affection for Big John, I had little respect for him.

While Big John was in jail, I became interested in astronomy, which was now my secret passion. I was fascinated with space travel and exploration, and I spent most of my precious spare time reading astronomy and science-fiction books. I lived vicariously through visionaries such as Jules Verne, who was later complemented by Arthur C. Clarke and my personal hero, Carl Sagan.

One day while riding in Big John's Cadillac, I took a chance and told him that I wanted to study astronomy when I grew up. Big John sniggered, "You're being foolish. There's no future in something as silly as astronomy. You need to put that out of your mind and concentrate on something you could earn a living at."

I countered that I *could* make money at it; I would just have to go to school longer.

He gripped the steering wheel, teeth bared and tension rolling off every muscle and fat roll. He didn't like the new me—the old me would never have argued with him. He shook his cantaloupe-size fist in my face and shouted, "If you want to see stars, I'll show you some stars! Now forget it. You're not going to be an astronomer. End of discussion. Got it?"

I got it, and I got a sickening feeling that the meat grinder of my childhood wasn't quite ready to spit me out yet.

Midway through the fall semester of my sophomore year of high school, Big John, who had been arrested and sent to jail again, got out once more, and his Mafia money enabled us to live like rich people. We moved to Long Island and I attended a nice high school like the ones I'd seen on television. However, my dad's gangster tactics made our home into a fucking nuthouse, and he terrorized me whenever his mood turned foul. I was thrilled for any excuse to escape, including a homecoming dance one Friday night, despite the fact that I didn't know how to dance and felt self-conscious.

The girls at the party looked pretty, but they were silly and tipsy; their permissive parents had allowed them to drink at home beforehand. My eyes veered toward a shy girl sitting on a chair, almost hidden from the crowd.

I thought she didn't look dangerous, and I liked her Italian beak nose; I floated over to her. "I'm Bob," I said and flinched; that sounded so common.

"I'm Elaine," she replied, and I relaxed a little; maybe simple introductions are common because they work. I grabbed a metal fold-up chair and sat down next to her.

When she wasn't staring at the gymnasium floor, I could see that Elaine had soulful brown eyes, accenting her lovely face that wasn't covered with makeup. As I asked her questions, she gave longer and longer responses, smiled more, and stopped tugging on the hem of her yellow skirt. After thirty minutes I mustered the courage to ask Elaine to dance. The band was playing "I Miss You So"; a slow one was easier for a novice like me. By the end of the song, I was plunged into the throes of new love for this delicate hummingbird. We talked all night and danced a few more times.

The following Sunday I took her to the movies, and afterwards she was my girlfriend. We were together every possible minute without raising my parents' suspicions. Elaine was my rock, my proof of beauty and integrity, and the calm I never got at home. It seemed odd I had to wait until I was fifteen to discover the peace and serenity that I could find only in her arms.

Near the end of the following summer, my father informed me that our family would go on vacation to a beach resort in Massachusetts. I fought to stay home; the idea of being separated from Elaine by hundreds of miles for several weeks was unbearable to me. Of course Big John won the battle, and I sulked in the backseat during the long car ride to Nantasket Beach.

We had only been there for three days, and I was missing Elaine. Big John was overbearing as always. I escaped our oceanfront condo and his bellowing voice and headed for the Nantasket pier. I planned to launch my tiny rowboat at the pier, hoping to peacefully click off the time until this imprisoning vacation was over and I could return to Elaine. However, Big John had alternate plans for me—and my face.

I was talking to a pretty girl near the launch dock when I saw him darting toward me. He had given me strict orders against flirting with girls. He was gritting his teeth and readying both his fists. Most of the time he was a gentle giant, but he also had a foul temper and was prone to violence.

Dad was strong, but I had speed on my side. I wasn't about to stand there and get my ass kicked. A walrus couldn't catch a fox. Watching his oncoming charge, I simply leaped over the pier railing and landed in the water twenty feet below.

"Get out of the ocean and into my damn car," Big John bellowed as I treaded water in the surf. I ignored him, just wanting to enjoy the warm sunlight at the pier. Suddenly his voice softened, "Bobby, please. Get into the car . . . please. And nothing will happen. Everything will be fine; we'll just talk. I promise." I acquiesced and trudged to his Cadillac.

That's when I learned that a gangster has no respect for his own word or anyone else's. As I closed the car door, his thick bicep punched me in the jaw. My head ricocheted against the passenger window and I tasted the metallic tinge of blood mixing with the salty remnants of ocean water. He started the car for home without a word. Something transformed in me in that moment—an assured knowing that he would never humiliate me again. Big John had battered me for the last time.

We were traveling about forty miles per hour, but I opened the door and tumbled out of the car onto the street. I rolled over several times, feeling the sharp gravel biting at my arms and stomach and through my pants. I heard the brakes screech, but Big John didn't stop. I managed to stand and, although dizzy and disoriented, ran like someone chasing freedom. I never looked back. I wanted that image to stay forever with Big John—me running away in his rearview mirror.

While Big John might have terrified the underworld, I was Fast Bob; I knew "you couldn't hit what you couldn't catch." I vowed that fat fuck would never catch me again.

If I had planned ahead, I probably would've gone home and gotten some food and an extra shirt before running away, but I knew that any hesitation, any procrastination, would only lead to additional humiliation. I stopped for a moment on the shoulder of the road on this narrow isthmus, breathing hard and looking at the road ahead and at Massachusetts Bay at both sides. In that moment, my problems transformed from getting beaten to death to starving to death. *Where would I eat and sleep?* I was penniless, so I hitchhiked to Long Island. I was glad I had kept Elaine secret from my parents. She didn't need gang-sters showing up on her doorstep, scaring her mother, and dragging her into Big John's underworld.

I threw pebbles at Elaine's window until I caught her attention. Thinking it was the neighborhood boys, she was about to yell until she saw me. She grabbed her jacket, threw a leash on the dog, and was out the door twenty seconds later. Half a block from her house in front of a creek that ran between two split-level homes, she turned to me. Tears welled in her eyes.

"Oh, Bobby! What happened?" She brought her hand to my chin, caressing me so carefully, then she leaned in and blew soft kisses.

I had a thousand different feelings in that moment. I was ecstatic to be free, exhausted, pissed that my so-called father had created this fucked-up life for me, and passionately crazy about this girl before me. All those emotions combined into a droll response. "Big John happened."

She brought out a lace handkerchief from her pocket, dipped it in the creek water, and wiped away the blood on my chin, elbows, shins, and countless other nicks. Biting her lip so that it almost bled too, she stayed silent for a long time, nursing all my Big John scars and the scrapes from my collision with the road.

"What will you do now?" she finally asked.

I grabbed her hands as the dog, her excuse to escape the house, nipped at my ankles, "I'm not going back. I'm a man now, and I'll act as such."

"Where will you stay?"

I didn't want her to worry, so I lied. "Oh, I have some old friends from the neighborhood. Their parents aren't around. I won't have any problems."

She nodded and hugged me for a long time, trying to make all the hurt go away. Off in the distance, we saw the front door of her house open and we had to say good-bye. She quickly kissed me and was gone.

God, I loved Elaine. I lived only for the moments I could spend with her. She kept me sane and grounded, and she gave me all the money she had; it was enough to keep me alive as I frantically looked for work. She went without lunch and the nice new things she could have bought with her babysitting money. She snuck me sandwiches and fruit, and I slipped into her house for a quick shower when her parents were working. Even then I had to be careful; her two annoying brothers would snitch to their parents if they knew. I wondered if her brother Tommy ever missed a couple shirts and great pair of jeans. I felt awful about asking Elaine for those favors, but during those days she taught me so much about love, caring, and unconditional giving—lessons I should have learned from my parents. I wanted to take care of her, protect her, and comfort her, not the other way around.

The job search wasn't going well; since I looked too young, no one wanted to hire me. For the first two months, I snuck into cars to catch a few hours of restless sleep in the backseat, always scared I would get caught.

One frigid night spent shivering and rubbing my numbed hands and feet convinced me I needed another way to sleep; only the six inches of snow shrouding the car that night saved me from frostbite. So afterwards I spent the fifteen cents I received daily from Elaine and bought fares on the rapid transit system.

Each night I boarded the elevated trains into New York City, where I had free access to the subway and could catnap two hours in one direction then return the opposite way, night after night, back and forth like some giant pendulum. The subway cars were mostly deserted during the night, carrying only swing-shift workers, drunks, and other sleeping teenage runaways. There was one danger with this nightly trek—too many aggressive perverts hit on me for sex. I worried about the cops too. I knew some were dirty and searching for me as a favor to Big John, who had me labeled as a runaway juvenile delinquent.

One night during my subway catnap, a teenager staggered aboard with his right eye ripped open. Blood gushed out of his nose and mouth, streamed down his chin, and pooled on his shirt. I ran over and helped him sit down next to me. He collapsed onto my shoulder, slipping in and out of consciousness. I held him in my arms, not knowing what the hell to do with him and trying to ignore that his blood was splattered across my only shirt.

I no longer felt like a kid forced into adult situations; I was now a man. For the first time in my life I recognized this strong compulsion to help endangered human beings, even strangers. Then I realized I was alone; I scanned the other faces in the subway car, and no one bothered to look at this poor soul.

The kid awoke twenty minutes later and began talking in a foreign language I couldn't understand. He looked Puerto Rican, and after several minutes of frenetic but groggy gesturing, I realized he wanted me to help him get home. The boy grimaced from the rocking motion and moaned every time the car stopped at a station. After two hours of switching subways and soliciting a translator, we got off. He needed a doctor but directed me to his home instead of to a hospital.

Blocks upon blocks, I carried him through a frightening part of New York City, past a huge dead dog getting devoured by rats and bums loaded on cheap booze and God knew what else. Countless dark buildings looked menacing in their bombed-out appearance. My patient gave me the sign language not to look anyone in the face. He then passed his hand in a cutting motion across his throat.

Oh my God. What the hell kind of combat zone have I gotten myself into now?

When we arrived at his building, I attempted to say good-bye, but he clung to my neck and began screaming. I didn't want to attract attention, so I leaned him on my shoulder, breathed deeply, and looked at the stairs. I was exhausted and doubted I possessed the strength to climb them alone, never mind lugging this boy with me. He needed me though, so I shrugged and began climbing five flights. We passed a five-year-old girl sleeping with a teddy bear on the third floor landing, and I tried to ignore the vile sewer stench that grew stronger as we climbed. When we got to his door, he gave it three giant kicks.

What the hell kind of knock is this? When the door opened, my heart fell into the ugly depths. Towering over me were four of the baddest, meanest, tattooed motherfuckers I had ever seen.

Before the door swung fully open, they knocked me to the floor and snatched my patient from my grasp. The fattest one had his foot poised over my face when the boy started screaming again. Whatever he said worked. At once they pulled me to my feet and hugged me. Once inside, the fat one got on the phone and called a brother who could speak English.

"*Gracias, señor*," said the accented, slightly tipsy brother through the telephone. "You help my brother, you're my brother. If you need help off-ing someone or ass-kicking, just call us, *hermano*, ok?"

Relieved that I wouldn't be leaving the apartment looking worse than the boy I had carried upstairs, I said I needed to go. He replied it was not safe for me in this part of town alone, so the four brothers walked with me to the subway station and handed me the best emblem of heartfelt thanks: a ten-dollar bill.

My outlook on life changed that evening. If not for the Good Samaritan money, I would not have had even the fifteen cents for the train to return to Elaine. When I arrived in Long Island, I promised her a nice dinner. She was shocked when we arrived at the local L&E Huts, a glorified White Castle hamburger joint, but after all her help keeping my spirit and body on speaking terms, she sure deserved it.

She had a forty-five-cent hamburger and I had a forty-nine-cent scrambled egg sandwich; we shared a Coke. The total bill came to a whopping $1.25.

I couldn't rent a room without money, and I looked so young the landlords said, "Why, you're only a school boy, sonny—go on, get out of here." But today I did have money, and I wasn't going to let this opportunity slip away without every effort to find my own bed.

In the local newspaper, I saw several rooms for rent. At the first two I tried, the owners just laughed at me. I got lucky with the third—a nearly blind old lady. I penciled in a thin mustache and wore a cap. The room had a soft, *horizontal* bed, and she was asking five dollars a week, so I handed over the Puerto Rican's bloody ten. I had been awake for three days and close to fainting from exhaustion. She gave me the key; I hustled her out, locked the door, and dove into bed. I slept thirty-four hours without even a pee run.

When I awoke I felt like King Kong. I was made anew, ready to conquer the world, even as I ignored my emaciated chest and hollowed eyes when I looked in the mirror. That day I spent ten hours canvassing countless restaurants for work: janitor, waiter, anything. Finally a dumpy little greasy spoon hired me as a dishwasher.

About a month later, I met Elaine after school and we went to the local pizza spot, filled with loitering teenagers and the aromas of yeasty dough and basil. She was trembling and covering her face with her hands, but I could not imagine what was wrong.

She grabbed my hand and placed it on her stomach, "I have not had a period for five months, and I feel kicking in my tummy!"

I felt transported to another planet. All of life changed in those few seconds, but I knew I'd be a better father than Big Jerk John. We talked and hugged and cried until the sun went down and the dinner crowd arrived, wanting their pizza and our table.

I propped my index finger beneath her chin and stared into her chocolate eyes, hoping she'd see my sincerity and feel safe. "We'll talk to your parents together tomorrow when you get out of school. They won't be quite so mad if we stand united."

Elaine stood up. "I best get going. My parents believe that good girls are home by sundown." She flashed me an ironic smile—the first one I had seen from her that day. She wiped her eyes with a red-and-white-checkered napkin and was gone.

When I arrived at her house the next afternoon, her driveway was packed with family cars. I stayed outside and cased the house like a good gangster son. After twenty minutes I saw Elaine fling open the door of her house and rush toward me; mascara ran down her cheeks, marring her sweet face.

I swept her into my arms, wiping away her black tears. "What the hell is going on?"

She looked up at me, appearing sad and lost. "I'm sorry. I told them and they called the entire family. My mom was so quiet and red-faced—I've never seen her like that. Dad said we were just two kids that needed to marry and have our baby. How are we going to do it?"

I leaned down and kissed her hair. "I have no idea." I felt guilty that I didn't have anything more encouraging to say. Only a few weeks earlier,

I was riding the New York City rails like some urban hobo; I wasn't even old enough to drive.

Walking into the house packed with relatives was a new experience, since I'd never had much family. Some were crying, others were hugging, and several were looking at me like I was a child rapist. I couldn't blame them; Elaine's parents had been kind to me, knowing I had a despicable family life.

Elaine's aunt pronounced that abortion was the only answer. I was mortified at the idea of an illegal, unsafe abortion that could harm my sweet Elaine and kill my child. A fire lit in my belly. I felt like a grown-up and didn't want these people making my choices and deciding my life.

Both Elaine and her mom, Georgianne, instantly recoiled from that suggestion, and Georgianne nixed it. She proposed adoption, which was better but still not an option either Elaine or I wanted.

At an impasse, Elaine's father spoke up. "I think we need to hear what these kids are feeling." Victor was rational, and I knew his perspective would help cut through the soap opera. He stood up, his nose inches from mine, and said, "Being a man and understanding how most men think, I'm sure Bob can't wait to get out of town so he can run away from this problem and on to another conquest."

I shook my head emphatically no. "You're wrong, Mr. Kruze. That's the last thing I want." I kissed Elaine's hand and held it against my heart. "I love Elaine, and I would never walk away—never! I want to marry Elaine and support our baby."

Still skeptical, Victor looked to his daughter. "Elaine?"

Elaine, still reeling from the abortion suggestion, needed some time to relax so that she could speak clearly. She whispered, "I love Bob and I want us to marry and raise our child together."

Vick continued, "Well, that's good enough for me if it's really what you both want." He looked at me. "We must have your parents' approval, and you've been estranged for almost a year. Bobby, they'll have to help you marry Elaine."

I detested the idea of asking Big John for anything, but I was no longer a kid and Elaine was definitely worth the risk. "I can and will do it, Mr. Kruze. That's a promise."

Elaine's mom, Georgianne, spoke up again. She was short, had lost most of her hearing, and had a fiery soul. "I can see my daughter loves you very much. However, I doubt we will ever hear from you again once you walk out that door."

"Elaine and I need a moment." I stood up, took Elaine's hand into mine, and led her onto the front porch. "Tell me from your heart what you want."

She held me tighter than I had ever been hugged and cried, "I want us to be a family together forever. Please Bob, please do it for us and our baby!"

Her passion settled it for me. I collected my twenty-seven-dollar paycheck on the last day at my dishwashing job and caught a Greyhound bus back to Boston. When I first spotted my parents' house, I noticed it looked as rundown as ever; their focus was always elsewhere—on alcohol, cigarettes, and whatever my dad did with his mob friends. I sank onto the concrete stoop, apprehensive about what lay ahead. I pictured Elaine's eyes, stood up, and knocked at their door three times. The door swung slowly open until it revealed me standing there.

Mom trembled in shock. As she started to collapse, I quickly reached out and grabbed her. She began sobbing, "You came back; you came back."

"Yes, Mom, I'm back and I need you."

Her eyes sharpened from their usual alcohol-induced glassiness, and she appeared alert. "Tell me what's wrong, Bobby. I will do anything to help you, but please don't run away again. It'll kill me, Bobby."

This last year almost killed me, Mom.

"Let me explain, and I pray you'll help me. My girlfriend, Elaine, in New York—I love her with all my heart—is pregnant and we're planning to marry."

After a long silence she blurted out, "I have to talk to your dad, but I don't want you to be here. I don't know what he'll do." She scanned the messy living room for options. "I know, hide in the closet when he comes in, and you can listen while I tell him all of this. If he gets crazy mad, we can wait until he goes into the bedroom; then you can run out the door."

Although this plan sounded nutty and inspired by bourbon, it seemed logical for my house. Countless times, Mom looked out the window for

Dad to drive up to the apartment complex; she kept hugging me, looking at me, and playing with my shirt collar. When she spotted him, she hustled me into the closet and covered me with a sheet. Despite the urgency, we were laughing at the inherent silliness, but I let her handle it her way.

Big John walked in and crossed over to the liquor cabinet. In a shaky voice Mom said, "Honey, I have a surprise for you."

He looked up from his scotch and water.

"Bobby came back home today."

There was a long pause. "What's the trouble?"

Mom recounted Elaine's pregnancy. He seemed pleased and not prone to start yelling or punching, so Mom called, "Bobby, come on out and talk to your dad."

Apprehensive, I poked my head out. He reached his hands to me and gave me a hug, nearly smothering me in his voluminous chest and strong biceps.

"Welcome back, son. I'm truly sorry for the way I handled everything at the pier."

The hard shell around my heart cracked slightly. I felt like the prodigal son. "It's okay, Dad," I said, although I knew deep down it wasn't. "It's behind us now."

He released me from his hug. "The past year was a nightmare for your mom. She cried all the time worrying about you."

That ignited a slight twinge of guilt that quickly was replaced by a sense of justice. I was happy to be home though.

—◆—

Our son, John, was born on July 17, 1953. Elaine's family stayed at our apartment for that week. During that time at least fifteen top Boston mobsters came to pay their respect to Big John's new grandson. Each gangster came to the crib, reached in, and touched the baby. They made the sign of the cross and then dropped wads of cash into the crib. Some of the code names written on the cash sounded like names from the children's books I would soon read to my new son. There was Mr. Moo, Mr. Hat, Pussy, Wimpy, Buster, and Mr. Waco.

The wads totaled two thousand dollars, a princely sum for Elaine's parents, who didn't understand why I wasn't proud of my father's business associates. I declined to explain.

Dad leased us a cozy apartment, bought us new furniture, and gave us a two-year-old Pontiac. I got a job as a painter and soon was foreman of a project to spray-paint the ceiling of a three-thousand-square-foot factory in Somersworth, New Hampshire.

As the months passed, Elaine grew more and more miserable living in Boston, away from her mom and large, loving family. The loneliness brought out a surprising Italian temper and razor-sharp tongue. Sometimes she could not resist snapping with unbelievably mean venom. Whenever she launched into her tirades, my reaction was to walk out the door and disappear for several days. I was young and stupid and knew no better way to react. To be fair, though, she was a great mother to our son and most times a great wife. And sometimes I was a real jerk.

That year when I was fifteen had been a hellish teeter-totter. It seesawed from poverty when my dad was in prison to riches when he came back home, from a grand vacation house overlooking the ocean to being homeless, from avoiding scary-guy sex to making love with my sweet Elaine. Along the way, I abandoned an abstract concept of character and proved myself to be resourceful and compassionate. And from it all, I emerged as a husband, a father, and my own man.

<hr />

A few years later, my dad was released yet again from prison (for holding the money that had been robbed from an armored truck) and was discovered in his Cadillac with two bullets in the back of his head. Someone had hid in his car and ambushed him. A few weeks later, the head of his partner, Wimpy Bennett, was delivered to his brother Walter at his pool parlor. When Walter searched for his brother's killer, he was murdered along with a third brother who had no involvement in the robbery or the aftermath. The Mafia was sending a message for all to beware of screwing up and bringing heat on it, chillingly known as the Black Hand.

My father's death flattened my mother's spirit for a long time afterwards. I was devastated but unsurprised. I grew up knowing my father wouldn't die in a bed. He was such a powerful man—but also a powerful force of nature. So many of the choices in my life had been either in support or in defiance of him. When he died, I felt strangely freed from his path and knew that my own journey was now finally about to begin.

In later years I witnessed the enormous love affair people have with the Mafia from the popularity of numerous Hollywood productions, including *The Godfather* and *The Sopranos*. Since I grew up in a Mafia family, I knew gangsters were only lowlife killers, no different from and no more glamorous than the drive-by gangbangers and terrorists who indiscriminately killed young men, women, and children for standing on the wrong street corner or wearing the wrong colors. For me, human lives were sacred. I valued our existence and wanted to do everything I could to preserve and prolong precious life.

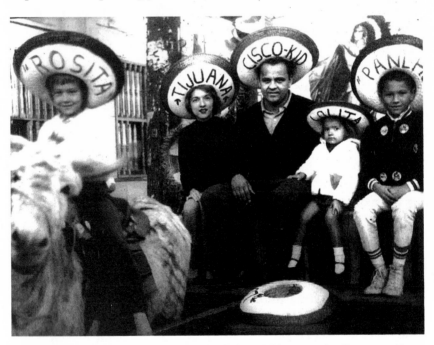

In 1962, soon after moving to California, Bob took his young family on vacation to Tijuana, Mexico.

CHAPTER 2

My Moment of Transformation

TEN YEARS LATER, ELAINE AND I WERE STILL MARRIED and still fighting. She still had a nasty mouth. I still had a penchant for leaving, and I still kept coming back because of her radiant spirit and our three adorable children—John, Lori, and our little Susan. During that time, we had switched coasts and moved to Los Angeles, where I settled into my career as a TV repairman. In our arguments, I admitted she was right about a few things: I was preoccupied with astronomy and obsessed with starting my own business. Ever since I was a little kid, forced into subservience by Grandma Witch and Big John, I had hated the idea of working for anyone else.

Those disagreements had led to our extended separation in the summer of 1965, which led me on a collision course with Professor Ettinger's *The Prospect of Immortality*. I had moved in with my friend Richard. His mother, Stella, was a wealthy and brilliant attorney, and she hoped I could keep Richard from drifting back to his heroin addiction. On the day I transferred my clothes to his plush apartment, I saw a birthday girl cutting her cake beside the swimming pool. She bewitched me with her hypnotic gaze and warm smile, looking yummier than the cake and reminding me of the legendary actress Ingrid Bergman.

The next morning I awoke from a peaceful sleep to the loud thud of a cannonball body hitting the water and a crescendo of laughter and screaming. I felt guilty, thinking my wife probably was not having a peaceful day with our small children. I peeked out and spied the birthday girl standing at the pool's edge. Every speck of her ravishing body not hidden by her lavender bikini evoked feminine tenderness; her breasts were the perfect size and slope, reminding me of a spectacular ski jump.

I quickly jumped into my swim trunks and proceeded out the door to join in the cannonball express. Three girls were at the far end of the pool. Instead of a thunderous entrance, I slipped in quietly and swam underwater toward the six tanned female legs.

When I arrived at the legs, I popped my head up out of the water, "Excuse me, girls, do any of you know Bob Nelson?"

With my sudden appearance, they looked at one another bewildered, shaking their heads. One finally said, "No, we don't know him."

I then asked, with a cheeky grin, "Would you like to meet him?"

I noticed the apartment manager, Angie, calling and waving for me to come over, gesturing to her newspaper. She had flirted with me before and was probably just jealous, so I ignored her since I was feeling some heady potential in the pool.

Even my Ingrid Bergman beckoned me. "Come on, Bob, and play cannonball with us."

But Angie insisted, "Come here, Bob; this is important." Her hand waved hurry, *hurry!*

I made an accounting of my dilemma: six eager eyes, three happy mouths, and six supple breasts versus Angie's hand holding a decidedly *unimportant* newspaper. My choice was clear, though. I reluctantly climbed out of the pool and splattered over to the concrete steps to see why she needed me so damned terribly much.

Angie looked up, her eyes coquettish. "Have you ever heard of freezing people a moment before their death and then many years later returning them back to life?"

I stared in disbelief at her words as the ground seemed to shift beneath me. My imagination stretched to its absolute mind-boggling limit.

"What kind of nonsense is this, science fiction?" I blurted.

Angie seemed exasperated with me. "No, this is for real. A Michigan physics professor has written a book titled *The Prospect of Immortality.*"

I grabbed her newspaper, slowly reading the article about Professor Robert Ettinger to soak up every precious word from those scant paragraphs—to force that knowledge into my brain, even by osmosis. I was shocked, and the three lovelies in the pool were completely forgotten.

Was it possible that death could be altered by this procedure? Could we really freeze people—and sometime in the distant future, wake them up?

I don't remember leaving the building or asking permission to take Angie's newspaper, but somehow I wound up in my car rereading the article again and again. I was entranced. That night I couldn't sleep and couldn't stop fantasizing that cryonics would change life and death on our planet. I felt transported, just as when I had heard in 1957 that the Soviets had launched *Sputnik* into orbit. Traveling to other worlds was now possible, adding decades to one's life was now possible, and seeing civilization hundreds of years after being born was now possible. That concept of limitless possibility left me dizzy.

The idea was at once preposterous and yet completely logical. But I couldn't make an evaluation about cryonics based on the filtered and simplified version written by a journalist. I needed to go to the source and read Professor Ettinger's book.

A week earlier I had signed a huge contract with a company called Nadel to repair all the damaged electronics they had bought and shipped from anywhere in the United States. It was quite an opportunity for me, and I was scheduled to start that next morning. But I was thinking of bigger issues than switches, wires, and transformers. I could only focus on the transformative power of the technology hinted at by that newspaper article.

I stopped by several bookstores on the way to my first sales meeting, but no one had yet received Professor Ettinger's book from the publisher. Finally, in the Yellow Pages I found a bookstore in Santa Monica that had just gotten the book, their shipment still unpacked.

I hated postponing such a good business opportunity, but I called Nadel and rescheduled our first sales meeting. I raced to the store to pick up the book and offered to pay them double, even triple, for a copy. I offered to help unpack, tempted to get on my knees and plead for this book. The guy at the counter thought I was a nutcase, so he went into the stockroom and returned several minutes later with a single copy of *The Prospect of Immortality*. Grabbing it from his hand, I began reading before reaching my car. I was enraptured from the first line in the preface written by legendary cryobiologist Professor Gene Rostand: "We are at last forced to concede the real possibility that the means for freezing and resuscitating human beings will one day be perfected, at however distant a time this may be."

What a strange choice of words. "We are at last forced to concede . . ."

I drove down Sunset Boulevard to the beach, gleaning more tidbits of precious information at each stoplight. I grabbed a blanket from my Porsche, looked for an isolated spot in the sand, and settled down to devour the book; spellbound, I lost all track of time. I read as the sun ascended far overhead, as the high tide forced me to scoot back a few feet, and until the dying twilight rendered further reading impossible. I closed the cover and stared at the book. It had crisp pages and a sharp binding in the morning; now it looked worn.

It is difficult to describe my reaction to Professor Ettinger's book—so much potential, so much hope was contained between the covers of this astounding book. For the first time in my life, I could see a bright light at the end of the tunnel of my existence, and the warmth of this light was very comforting indeed.

I envisioned governments and billionaires from around the world clamoring to fund cryonics suspension research. Professor Ettinger would be deluged with grants to support this life-giving science. I looked out at the Pacific Ocean and could almost visualize on the horizon a spaceship from another galaxy, gifting us mortals with information that would save billions of research dollars and centuries of research—catapulting our world eons ahead with scientific knowledge.

I was convinced that what Ettinger proposed would be done immediately. I foresaw the Soviets, who had challenged us to a race to the moon, challenging us to a new race—to break the "biological ice barrier." Cryonics intersected my love of astronomy, as I understood that suspended animation would be a necessary ingredient for long-term space travel. It would allow people to stay dormant for months, even years, without overwhelming life support requirements. When they arrived at their distant planet, they could then be revived. With cryonics, we could travel to far-away solar systems and galaxies. Professor Ettinger's book was embellished with stardust, and that stardust had forever touched me.

My mind was inexorably bent toward cryonics and this new way of looking at death. For if a person can be revived, then he had never actually died. This is probably the most misunderstood aspect of cryonics suspension. Once a person is dead, he is dead. Nothing can bring a dead body back to life. But death does not happen in an instant; we travel a long journey to the land beyond the veil. Along that path, we pass through a complicated biological sequence as blood stops flowing, chemical reactions halt, electrical impulses stop, and there is no life force to prevent the decay. By lowering the body temperature at an early stage of the dying process (that is, clinical death), we slow down the journey and stop the dying progression, thereby keeping the patient from ever reaching the stage of complete irretrievable death. Freeze the person and stop the dying.

Cold slows down the biological clock; the colder the environment, the slower the clock. So at liquid nitrogen temperatures (-320°F; for comparison, 200 proof alcohol freezes at -173°F), time practically ceases to exist. These slowed chemical reactions are governed by the third law of thermodynamics. And through the years, I've discovered that people's responses to cryonics are governed by Newton's third law of motion: For every action, there is an equal and opposite reaction. As much as I love the potential and hope provided by cryonics, there are people who equally loathe the concept that cryonics can ever be a reality.

By altering our concept of death—that dying might be postponed hundreds of years—cryonics circumvents centuries of religious faith and beliefs that have been embraced for millennia. But life has a precedent of breaking such traditions of human behavior. This change is the natural order of life; it keeps happening again and again. And the privilege of witnessing such evolution and revolution is one of the primary and primal reasons I love being alive and why I want to stay alive for as long as I possibly can.

Sitting in the sand with a pink-and-orange sky before me, I wondered if I might be mentally unbalanced in this immediate and overwhelming fascination with the potential created by freezing people. I couldn't rationalize how obsessed I had become with this book while everyone else seemed more concerned with the price of gasoline.

To test my judgment, I returned to the Santa Monica bookstore a week later and purchased three more copies of Professor Ettinger's book, and then I pondered the people in my life that I considered to be the most intelligent and open-minded. The first was the Duke family, with whom I had lived as a renter for about three years.

The next person was my roommate's mother and a brilliant attorney, Stella Gramer.

The last victim was Paul Porcasi, who was an official with the Mensa society, an organization requiring members to have an IQ in the top 2 percent of the population.

I asked them to read *The Prospect of Immortality* and give me their opinion. Three for three, they agreed with me and found it logical and reasonably presented. Stella, in her late seventies, was prepared to sign up at once for her own suspension. She reasoned that if the procedure didn't work, she would simply remain dead. Paul agreed to help establish a legal organization to support freezing research and to publish a newsletter to educate the public about this fascinating new science.

Backed by their support, I felt assured I was thinking sensibly. The next couple of months were spent in an intellectual stasis, anxiously waiting to find someone that knew more about cryonics, and I was undeterred by the seeming indifference of the rest of the world.

I wasn't the saucer chaser or the self-taught pseudo-scientist. I needed some proof of concept. Even though I was young, with many years of life still before me, I knew that no one would emerge from suspended animation within my lifetime. Sure we could freeze people and leave them in liquid nitrogen indefinitely, but I needed some assurance, something more than faith, that reanimation truly did lie at the other end of the cryonics tunnel.

And I found that proof in the most unlikely place.

A few months after reading the book, I was still floundering, unsure if cryonics would dim from my consciousness or where it might lead. I was with my two daughters, Lori and Susan, absorbed in their universe of wide-eyed child discovery and worrying they would run off, so I brought them to a pet store because Susan loved the puppies.

At the checkout counter, hanging on a rack for last-minute purchases was a cellophane-wrapped package with giant red letters: Just ADD WATER. WATCH THEM COME TO LIFE.

As Lori wandered off to look at bunnies, I just stood there staring as the implications slowly washed over me. Susan saw it too and put a chubby finger on the red lettering. She sounded out the words.

"See . . . mon-kees." She looked up at me with big eyes. "Sea monkeys? That's funny."

"Yeah," I replied only half listening, concentrating too much on the fine print. "Yeah!" I repeated, more excited. I grabbed five packages and plopped them down on the counter. "When we go to your mom's, let's do a science experiment." I looked over my shoulders, scanning the aisles for Lori. "C'mon, c'mon," I hustled the kids out with the same excitement I'd often seen in them. I wanted to see the promised illustrations in action.

I raced back to Elaine's house with the kids, and she was gracious enough to let me set up in her kitchen. Lori grabbed a glass of water, while I ripped through the cellophane and tore open the Sea-Monkeys packet. A few particles of the beige powder went airborne, dancing in the golden light of late afternoon that streamed through Elaine's windows. I slowly, carefully, almost grain by grain, poured the powder into the glass of water.

We leaned in; Lori, Susan, and I knocked heads. Elaine stood back with an amused smile she reserved just for me.

Slowly, as if on command, little brine shrimp answered the curtain call. They emerged from tiny eggs and started swimming in the water. I beckoned Elaine to come over and see the sea monkeys for herself.

She crossed the kitchen and looked down on the glass, running her hand through Susan's hair. "Hmm, is that kind of like yeast?"

I felt light-headed. "Yeast? What do you mean?"

Elaine grabbed a foil package from a cupboard. "Yeast. It sits on a shelf until you need it; add water and sugar to wake them up. . . ." Her voice trailed off.

My mind started swimming again. That day, I witnessed suspended animation at work in single-celled microscopic yeast and this higher-order animal. Granted, these were just shrimp, not anywhere near as complex as a human, but they held possibility and hope in their random swimming. Their life had been suspended until my kids and I created the environment they needed to be reanimated. I was giddy. I now had my answer; I now had my proof.

I planted a big kiss on Elaine, probably an inappropriate kiss, considering our separate living arrangement, and floated out into a moonless night. I looked up at the twinkling stars and wondered which ones were now within reach.

~

There are actually many examples of suspended animation in nature. In southern Alaska, at the base of the White Horse Mountains, there is a snake that routinely undergoes a freezing phenomenon that is spectacularly enchanting to witness.

These snakes gather in autumn to breed, coming to a barren meadow by the thousands in their mating frenzy. After their annual breeding is complete, the snakes normally return to their underground homes to hibernate for the long, cold Alaskan winter.

Sometimes, sudden blizzards will capture thousands of these snakes before they can retreat to the safety of their burrows. Unprepared for the harsh icy grip of winter, the snakes are caught mid-slither and frozen solid in every imaginable configuration, their vast number extending to the horizon. They are then covered with several feet of winter's snow and will stay entombed for several months until surrendering to the warming rays of the spring.

An enchanting spectacle follows when the snow gives way to the first tender rays of spring's warmth. Winter's frigid grip begins to lessen its hold on these frozen lovers, slowly at first, then accelerating to where the snow melts, revealing its precious encased cargo.

During those first moments of sunlight, I would wonder if these frozen snakes covering a vast field were able to sustain and endure. And then the magic starts. One lone creature crosses back across that frozen chasm between life and nonlife, wriggling and squirming against months of lethargy. After about an hour of sunlight, dozens, hundreds, and then several thousands of the frozen snakes give a slight tremble.

Over the next hour, the entire mass of snakes shows a sustained quiver. Soon after, one by one, they begin to slither away—to return to their breeding ground the following year and perhaps once again get caught up in a winter wonderland.

That life can be frozen and arrested for long periods of time, and then resume when returned to a more favorable environment, is part of nature's design to save species from certain death. Humanity is now awakening to the reality that we too can use this gift of low-temperature biology. We can save and prolong the precious life of people who choose to take that chance on future technology.

CHAPTER 3

A TV Repairman Takes the Reins

A MONTH LATER, I WAS STOPPED IN TRAFFIC on the freeway, listening to Tony Bennett's "If I Ruled the World," when the DJ interrupted, speaking in a sarcastic tone. "If any of you listeners out there don't like the idea of dying someday, just call Helen Kline and get yourself invited to the first meeting of the Life Extension Society," he said. I turned up the volume and grabbed pen and paper from the glove box. "They believe that if you get your body frozen, then someday you can come back to life. Just imagine what a gas it'll be to see how much the world has changed in the next couple hundred years."

I nearly rear-ended the car in front of me. That DJ never realized the impact of his playful announcement on people's lives. I decided to attend this meeting and do whatever I could to support their goals.

In Los Angeles on May 13, 1966, I attended California's first LES meeting. As I got out of my Porsche, I spotted a ghostly house that reminded me of the Norman Bates house on the top of the hill in the movie *Psycho*. Chills coursed up my spine. However, not being superstitious, I just grinned at the ominous start of the evening and wondered what other surprises awaited me as I climbed the long stairs to Helen's door.

An elderly lady with an angelic smile greeted me at the entrance. We introduced ourselves and, strangely, I felt somehow connected to her. Helen looked worn out; she had a pronounced hump on her back and thinning gray hair. Helen's lips were pale, and her complexion was ashen white. She was also very thin, a side effect of the severe lung cancer that was slowly stealing away her life. She carried a huge wad of paper towels in her right hand and consistently coughed into it.

Through it all, she wore a radiant smile and a bright flowery dress and adorned herself with countless bracelets and a clunky necklace. Her sparkling eyes conveyed this beautiful lady's fighting spirit as she projected an energy comparable to a wildfire. She was not going to give up the ghost without a fight.

Single-handedly, she had brought together people who embraced Professor Ettinger's book and had gotten this meeting publicized on the radio. A frail little old lady had pulled off California's very first meeting to promote cryonics.

This meeting was nothing like I had imagined. There were no scientists in white lab coats, no businessmen wanting to capitalize on this profound event. With so many elderly people, this appeared to be an old-timers' storytelling group. I could see this was far from a scientific group of actual researchers but instead people who loved the idea of extended life. For me its purpose was tantamount to the first landing of an alien spaceship, intent on delivering control of aging and human immortality.

Professor Ettinger's book stirred up a fire in all of us. We looked at one another with the same expectant expression, gauging the hidden wisdom each might extol. Everyone's searching gaze communicated the same thought: Was this real?

I studied the other participants. Russ Stanley was a tall, thin, elderly man. He slouched over at the neck when he talked to me. He had an uncomfortable habit of getting his face close to mine as he spoke, and I could feel the spray on my face. Mixed with the saliva, however, was an encyclopedic knowledge of cryonics history from one of the world's most enthusiastic advocates.

"All human beings are on a sojourn here on Earth," he told me. "The most important part of this journey is to discover the revelations given to mankind by the Creator. Suspended animation is one of these great gifts."

Russ played an audiotape of Professor Ettinger's appearance on the *Johnny Carson Show* with Zsa Zsa Gabor. It was not easy for the physicist, since Johnny was poking fun and Zsa Zsa was injecting a sexy element into the mix. Nevertheless, he sounded brilliant. I'd not heard him speak before, and the professor's passion and eloquence intensified my belief in low-temperature biology.

"This science is no different than any other discipline of technology," Russ continued. "Human beings have advanced in every branch of science, and we continue to discover better ways. That will never change. We will continue to progress up and up and up forever—that will never change!"

Hearing Russ voice our shared philosophy, I knew I had found my people. I felt an immediate connection with this meeting's participants.

Several college students were present, including Dennis Guiley, who, from what I overheard, knew a lot about cryonics suspension. I wandered over and asked, "How will science improve human suspension?"

Dennis waved that off as he wove his fingers through his dreadlocks. "I don't really care about that; I'm more interested in the religious ramifications. I think we should first consider the effect on future world history rather than lab research."

I nodded, chagrined. Dennis had an infuriating mind-set: no chutzpah, only deep, mind-altering discussions. I was frustrated—I wanted action and I wanted it now! I also found myself in the unexpected position of being among the most knowledgeable people at the meeting, since I had read Professor Ettinger's book along with years of astronomy society articles.

Dick Jones was an attractive, articulate, middle-aged gentleman with a smiling face that made me want to laugh with him. Dick told me he had visited Michigan and met Professor Ettinger and likened the professor to Alexander Graham Bell or Thomas Edison. In time we became good friends, and he gave me passes to his comedy appearances with his partner, Jenna McMahon. They had written countless episodes for *The Carol Burnett Show* and won several Emmys.

I strolled over to a striking redhead, about forty years old, and my eyes kept veering toward her cleavage. Marcelon Johnson was an intelligent lady who impressed me with her broad knowledge. "As research continues, we should expect slow but steady advances as science freezes more biological organisms successfully. To not want it, I can understand. But not to see its inevitability, I cannot understand."

After several rounds of Pepsis and tea sandwiches, Marcelon called everyone together and suggested we accomplish some business. She asked if anyone knew the legalities of forming a nonprofit group to support low-temperature biology. I stuck my hand up and responded that my dear friend and attorney, Stella Gramer, likely would guide us around any legal minefields.

As we were concluding, Helen answered a knock at the door.

Dr. Renault Able had arrived.

His singular appearance commanded our attention; we just stared with our mouths agape. Dr. Able glided across the foyer, preparing to hold court. He wore diamonds, rubies, and sapphires on almost every finger, elevator shoes, and a suit that looked spun with magical silk. He had intense eyes and extremely thin lips, the whole effect reminiscent of Batman's nemesis, the Joker.

He spoke with a high-pitched voice and the showy, flowing gestures of an interpretive dance performer. "I have an interest and willingness to act as this group's official medical doctor. I must depart forthwith to perform a very lengthy surgery, so I must take my leave at once. Nevertheless, I wanted to grace this organization with my appearance and voice my consent to be counted as a member." With that, he proffered his business card, turned around, and sauntered out. Overcome with curiosity I ventured outside to see if his exit would be as dramatic as his entrance. He didn't disappoint; he stepped into a gleaming Rolls-Royce and drove away.

That meeting was quite remarkable, considering it attracted such a diverse mix of people. It made sense though. Despite our differences, we all will die, and we all wish to preserve the fragile strings keeping us tethered to this life.

Fate touched me on the shoulder that night, and four weeks later I was elected president at our second meeting. I felt quite humbled by this responsibility bestowed upon me. These people felt that I, a TV repairman, was worthy of directing this very important mission. In that moment, I found the legacy of my life.

I responded that I was willing to accept the responsibility until a more-qualified professional became available. All I had to do was figure out how to defeat death—and convince the world to accept it.

Several months later I incorporated the nonprofit Cryonics Society of California after a visit from CSNY (Cryonics Society of New York) president Curtis Henderson and its secretary, Saul Kent. CSNY had existed for a year, and we adopted its infrastructure. Saul and Curtis gave us an enormous education on cryonics and advised us to find a cooperating mortuary along with medical and hospital officials that would respect a patient's dying wish for interment. They were so helpful in getting the CSC started, and I have been indebted to them ever since.

I was elected president of the CSC; Dick Jones was secretary, and Marcelon Johnson was treasurer. During our third meeting at Helen Kline's home, Dr. Able surfaced again. We were delighted to see a medical doctor, and this time he said he could stay awhile. After we briefed him on the developments of the past three months and he discovered that I was president, he expressed his displeasure that an ordinary engineer was presiding over such a controversial group.

I took a deep breath, bracing myself for his reaction. "You have been misinformed, Dr. Able. I am not an engineer; I am a TV repairman."

Hearing this information, he went ballistic; his face turned as purple as his amethyst cufflinks. "I really must insist that someone with respectable credentials lead the society."

I smiled. I was fine with having a new leader. "Whom would you suggest direct our group?" I looked around the room. "Russ Stanley?"

He was immediately dismissed.

"How about Dennis Guiley?"

"A college student? Of course not," snapped Dr. Able.

A tiny smile flashed across my face. "Then that only leaves one logical person to lead our group, which is you, Dr. Able. Would you be so kind as to accept this role?"

Now his face turned from amethyst to aubergine. Obviously he would not subject his practice to the potential ridicule. Dr. Able stood up and paced back and forth, saying nothing.

He abruptly spun on his heel and announced, "I must leave. I will contemplate the necessary steps to address this situation. A television repairman as president of this organization is quite simply unacceptable."

With that, Dr. Able left and never attended another meeting. He phoned us occasionally and reiterated his willingness to help, but he still felt embarrassed by the society's choice of president.

Once we received our corporate approval and nonprofit status, Stella Gramer gave us a suite of offices in Westwood, California. Over the next six months, we appeared on several radio and television programs promoting cryonics and enlisted a prestigious scientific advisory board. All those tasks were to create the infrastructure for the action I so strongly craved.

⚫︎‿⚫︎

Being elected president of the CSC was both humbling and ennobling. Before the first meeting, I didn't think I was qualified even to attend, yet they had placed the entire operation in my inexperienced hands.

The honor brought me directly into the path of Professor Robert Ettinger. Once the CSC had raised enough funds, we petitioned Professor Ettinger to travel to California from Michigan and speak to our group about his thesis of extended life.

I was nervous about meeting the man who had changed the trajectory of my life. Never before had I so keenly felt the invisible cloak of my TV repairman job upon me. I worried that, like Dr. Able, he would find me wholly unsuitable.

Before Professor Ettinger arrived, I waited in Helen's living room. Nearby there was a huge table with juices, doughnuts, and apples, but I couldn't eat anything. I saw him enter, and since I'd always imagined him in a lab coat, his fine tailored suit was initially disconcerting. But it was a moment that will live in my memory for all time. How often does a person meet his hero?

Professor Ettinger had a commanding presence. When we shook hands, I felt this electric anticipation, and I hoped he didn't notice my sweaty palms. His eyes were striking; they were friendly but showed a sharp awareness that noticed every detail. I knew I couldn't participate in deep intellectual discussions about the intricacies of biophysics and cryonic research—at least not yet. We shared the same passion though, the same keen desire to move science out of the sterile confines of the laboratory and into the messy surroundings of life and death.

This brilliant physicist was a revelation. I learned a great deal from listening to him speak at the meeting. He had a way of simplifying complex concepts so that the layman could easily comprehend, and he did so eloquently. I later parroted many of his conceptualizations during TV and radio interviews.

He stayed as a guest in my home and addressed our group twice during his five-day visit. I realized how much we shared; he was called Bob by his friends and also married to an Elaine. In those few precious days, a complete metamorphosis occurred in my life. I was set free by Ettinger's and my shared love of science and life. It now seemed okay to reach for the moon.

From that initial meeting, we forged a lifelong friendship that continued to his *clinical* death in 2011. He was a university physics and astronomy professor. My stepfather had cared nothing about astronomy and had scolded me for my interest. This antithesis of Big John was now the role model of my life; he understood and encouraged every goal I set. The "father of cryonics" became my second father. And that really was our relationship throughout the forty-five years I knew him. This scientist never considered me inadequate or found anything wanting in me. I brought him my successes and my failures, and he helped me with them all.

During that visit to CSC, Professor Ettinger and I went together on a talk show with Joe Pyne. The man had a reputation for being rude and confrontational, and I felt nervous and unprepared.

Pyne stayed true to style and opened with a bang. He looked at me and said, "Mr. Nelson, I want you to explain who gives you the right? By whose authority do you think you can go around freezing people?"

Wide-eyed, I sat on the couch, flustered and flummoxed, and tried to compose something coherent.

Professor Ettinger leaned forward and intervened. "What credentials are required for anyone to freeze people, including me? What credentials are needed for extended life?"

Gratitude, relief, and respect flooded over me. Taken aback by Ettinger's measured response, Pyne then settled into a more cordial interview.

One evening during Ettinger's visit, we met with some medical professionals. A few were supportive but most were opposed, and we debated with one particular doctor at length. Finally, he said, exasperated, "You just can't change the world."

Professor Ettinger replied, "The hell I can't. I already have."

I turned to look at him, this man I had idolized, and realized he was right. A simple book, if it contains a radical and logical thesis, can change the world.

My wife Elaine and I had reconciled since our last extended break, but she was struggling to show enthusiasm for this strange twist I brought into our lives. Nevertheless, she offered her hospitality to Professor Ettinger during his stay. Before he returned to Michigan, he thanked Elaine and in parting said, "I'll see you again. If not in a year—well—in a thousand years."

— ❧ —

Cryonics was uncharted territory, and deciding what path CSC should take was crucial to its long-term success. Some cryonics groups were focusing on gaining membership; others were preparing storage for the expected flood of frozen patients.

I figured that if doctors were ever going to revive a frozen patient, we needed to protect the patient from damage caused by freezing. I decided that aggressive research would be our first priority.

Curtis Henderson and Saul Kent, the directors of CSNY, visited us in LA and arranged a meeting with Robert W. Prehoda, a medical researcher and prolific author studying cryobiology.

Meeting Robert at his home in Encino, California, was one of the most influential and informative conversations of my life. He was an expert in reduced metabolism and gave me a crash course in the underlying physics of cryonic freezing. Over the next several months, I went to college in his living room, and the coursework cemented my hope. I learned that on the evolutionary tree, man is not far from many natural hibernators.

I wrote Professor Ettinger about Robert and he wrote back that, yes, he knew of Robert's work but didn't have much respect for the man's character. Robert had praised *The Prospect of Immortality* after its initial release; however, he retreated from his original support after the scientific community disputed Ettinger's thesis. I saw Professor Ettinger's point but felt that Robert was too valuable and accepted him into the CSC.

I scavenged through Robert's brain for every morsel of information about the leaders in low-temperature biology. Slowly we established a

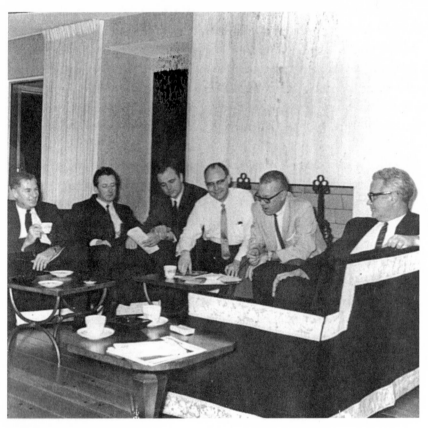

CSC Scientific Advisory Council

bond, although he knew I was mainly after his knowledge and I knew he was interested in the potential dollars CSC could deliver from research grants. We had a mutually beneficial, though not particularly affectionate, relationship.

Robert created collaborations with other scientists working in reduced-metabolism research. Two months later, Robert set up a meeting at his home. Five colleagues were interested in forming a scientific advisory council for CSC because of the research's potential for groundbreaking discoveries. CSC would provide funding, and Robert would help apply for grants.

The council was happy to provide research into human suspended animation but wanted no part in actually freezing anyone. If the CSC did freeze someone, the affiliation would be irrevocably dissolved. At the end of our meeting, we all felt we had achieved a monumental step forward.

That evening, I went home and told my wife the news. I was still giddy and amazed that I, a nonscientist without a college degree, was collaborating with scientists in such a revolutionary field. I had come so far from my days as a homeless teenager and wanted Elaine to be proud of me. Ever since I had moved back home, she had kept herself involved with the children and firmly disconnected from cryonics.

"What do you think?" I prodded after I told her about the advisory council.

Elaine bit her lip. "Well, it helps, I suppose. I guess it sounds more respectable now than one of those groups obsessed with flying saucers or life on other planets." She picked up Lori's ripped book bag. "But truly, Bob, who cares? Will it fix your daughter's backpack? That's what I'm concerned about. I tried calling you at work a dozen times today, and you weren't there earning a paycheck."

"I had more important things to do than fixing someone's TV set. Don't you understand the potential of what we're doing?"

"I understand that we could become destitute. It's almost like a cult. You moved back home a few months ago, but are you really part of this family?"

Feeling equal measures of anger and guilt, I struck back, "Of course I am. Everything I do with cryonics is for our children—so that they can have a longer, better life. My parents thought I was stupid to want to reach for the stars. John, Lori, and Susan will know different because of the example I set."

Elaine wouldn't back down. "Don't give me that. You're not with your kids. When you're not at work, you're there. When you should be at work, you're there. When you're at home, you're on the phone all the time. I even had to arrange a special code with my friends just so I would know they're calling. And honestly, all this cryonics stuff is weird—just plain weird."

I stormed outside and collapsed onto the porch steps. If I couldn't win the heart and mind of my own wife, then what prayer did I have for convincing the rest of the country?

One day in December 1966, a phone call made me realize that word of our exploits and our lofty goals had spread far beyond what I had anticipated.

"Hello," said a sweet-sounding woman, "I am an associate of the Walt Disney studio. Are you the group involved in suspended animation?"

Walt Disney? This call was huge. My mind started to race around her motivations—did she want to produce a film? Was Walt Disney interested for himself? I had heard he was close to death. . . .

"Yes, ma'am," I managed to stutter out.

"Wonderful. I'm trying to get some information. How many people have been frozen? Where is your facility? What doctors are involved?"

My heart sank; I couldn't offer anything substantive. "Ma'am, we are still exploring the potential of this forward-looking science. No one has been frozen, and there is no cryogenic facility. We are in scientific collaborations with two medical doctors, Dr. Dante Brunol and Dr. Renault Able." I summarized their credentials and our work with the advisory council.

"Thank you very much. You've been quite helpful."

"Wait," I said, but the phone call was over. I stared at the receiver for a long time, trying to process what the woman's motivations had been and frustrated that I didn't have more encouraging results to provide.

I never learned if she had called because of personal interest by Walt Disney, and I never heard from her again. I also never heard if anyone else in the cryonics community was contacted. As far as I know, this lone phone call is the entire basis for the urban legend that Disney was frozen. His family denies that he had any interest in cryonics, but I still like to believe that the curiosity of a visionary of Disney's caliber was piqued by the concept of suspended animation. If he had been the first person frozen, I am sure the trajectory of cryonics would have been far different and many of the later sad events would not have occurred.

Nevertheless, in December 1966, cryonics was a bright golden vista with limitless possibilities on the horizon. About one month after that phone call, the CSC, with an inexperienced TV repairman at the helm, accomplished the pioneering feat of freezing the first human by cryonic suspension.

CHAPTER 4

Man Becomes Immortal

IN EARLY 1967, ROBERT PREHODA AND I WERE at our offices in West-wood, working on a list of promising foundations that would accept our research proposals. I received a call from a funeral director; he spoke fast and sounded desperate.

"This is Mr. Clark from the Stedford Mortuary in Glendale," he said. "We have a gentleman giving us just a god-awful time about wanting to freeze his father, who's very close to death. I have no idea what in the world he's talking about, and he won't leave until I arrange to have his father frozen." He exhaled through the phone. "Would you please talk to him? Maybe you can make some sense."

The man in the mortuary office was Norman Bedford, and his father, Dr. James Bedford, wanted to be frozen and suspended. I asked Mr. Clark to hold on for a moment while the shock subsided enough so I could speak sensibly. Then I said, "Mr. Clark, my name is Robert Nelson. I'm the president of the Cryonics Society of California, and I think I can help you."

I wrote down his phone number and promised I'd call him right back. I dropped the phone back in its cradle and realized that I had five minutes to accomplish what I couldn't in the past six months—convince Robert that a successful freezing would catapult our goals and outreach forward by years. With this decision, we would be crossing Caesar's Rubicon. We would be staking our reputation and legacy on an untried, and by many accounts unscientific, scheme.

After thinking for a few minutes and mentally compiling a list of a hundred tasks, I decided just to be truthful and gauge his reaction.

I walked into his office and said, "That call was from a mortuary in Glendale. The funeral director has a client who wants his father's body frozen. Apparently the man's near death."

"Oh my God," Robert said. He dropped his pen and stared at me over his reading glasses. "I hope you're not going to do it! We haven't perfected a protocol yet, and you know damn well it's going to piss off the advisory council."

I needed time to consider the ramifications and ask Professor Ettinger for guidance, but Robert's stern rebuke told me I had to think fast. "How about I invite this young man for a talk tomorrow before we draw any conclusions?"

Robert's face lit up, since I'd guaranteed he'd be included. He agreed to meet Norman and offered his elegant home in Encino. I called the Stedford Mortuary back, and Mr. Clark handed the phone to Norman. I assured him that he had called the right people to fulfill his father's wishes. We agreed to meet at Robert's house the following morning at 9:00 a.m.

I called Professor Ettinger that evening, excited that I could give such good news to this man who had changed my life. I left the decision up to him.

"This is wonderful news and the most exciting development to date," he said. "This will open the field to the entire world—someone of Bedford's caliber, a university psychology professor, will be magic. We need to do this if we possibly can." Such is the brilliant logic of my hero friend and father of the cryonics movement. He advised me to proceed with coordinating the men and necessary equipment for this historic event.

I replied, "I'm concerned though. We're likely to lose our scientific advisory board."

Professor Ettinger wasn't worried. "If you're truly ready, then you should proceed anyway. This is far more important. Freezing the first man will be a major accomplishment, garnering worldwide attention. You'll probably get these guys back afterwards."

I agreed with him. Indeed, such a profound success would eclipse any problems that could arise from losing the board's support. I threw out another concern: "Prehoda's worried that the protocol is too damaging to the brain."

"I've examined the details. It's close enough. I'll ship the cardiac compression machine you'll need during the perfusion operation." He paused for a moment and his voice sounded more reflective. "You're starting an amazing voyage."

Professor Ettinger asked me several questions about the intended doctor, the chemicals, and the immediate storage.

I hung up, feeling assured. I was confident enough to believe that it could be done and optimistic enough to not understand why it shouldn't. Through his approval, Ettinger decided that CSC would freeze the first human being.

The next morning I sat on the sofa in Prehoda's parlor, thinking about questions and strategies for the meeting. Dr. Dante Brunol had arrived; he was a biophysicist working on a perfusion procedure—a step-by-step guide for preserving a human being. I felt his presence lent much-needed medical credibility as well as another friendly opinion on human freezing.

Soon after Brunol, Norman Bedford rang the doorbell. He was about thirty, with a beard and close-cropped dark hair, but the intensity on his face was almost scary. Since his father was dying and he was exploring quite an exotic option, I was sure that exacerbated his high-strung personality. I began by asking Norman about his expectations.

Flush-faced and frenetic, Norman fired out questions: "My father wants to be frozen and that's it. Can we do it? What needs to be done?" He wagged his finger in my face. "My father is near death, and I don't have time to deal with anyone who's going to drag their feet."

I tried to ease Norman's fears; the man's hands just would not stop twitching. "You're talking to the right people. Your father will be the first case, but CSC has invested a lot of research into cryonics; we're prepared to do it right."

He seemed to relax a little. He said his father had read Professor Ettinger's book, discussed longevity in his classes, and determined to be frozen when he died.

I decided to plunge further: "We need your father's written authorization before we can do anything."

"That won't be a problem, considering it was his idea anyway."

Then there was the necessary funding to provide for all the supplies. I launched into a long list of chemicals and equipment necessary to complete the procedure, along with a temporary dry-ice storage container for the patient and, finally, a second container for the patient, to be filled with liquid nitrogen for the duration of the suspension. There was also the problem of where the liquid nitrogen container would be stored.

Norman had been writing all this down, his hand flying across his notebook. He leaned in to speak, his nose about four inches from mine. "Can the society provide all those requirements? If you can't, then I'll find someone who'll get what you can't."

"I believe we can," I replied, using my soothing fatherly voice. "But we'll need a cooperating doctor at the moment of death."

"Just give me whatever papers you need and my dad will sign them," Norman responded. "As for money, my father has three hundred thousand dollars in a foundation for cryobiological research, and I am director of that foundation. Will that be enough to cover the expenses of my father's freezing?"

Robert's eyes widened, and a slight smile appeared; that much money definitely got his attention. I requested that Norman allow a private moment among my colleagues.

We excused ourselves into the kitchen, and I asked Dr. Brunol, "What do you think?"

He almost jumped into my arms while replying "Yes." I smiled and then looked at Robert, suggesting that he could act as an advisor. I could see he was anxious to perform the suspension. I reminded him that we'd lose our scientific advisory council.

"Well," Robert shrugged, thinking about the ramifications, "perhaps for just a little while."

I could not believe our luck. Not only had we secured Robert's support, but he had agreed to help organize the actual freezing. I was giddy;

here was the action I so craved, and I felt absolutely confident that I could engineer this procedure.

I spent the next several days constructing the dry-ice box, coordinating people's schedules, and purchasing syringes and the chemicals with the proper purity. It seemed incredible that with such seemingly mundane tasks, we were preparing to freeze the very first human being for future reanimation.

Dr. Brunol had given me a checklist of chemicals and equipment needed for his perfusion procedure. Although the specifics are certainly outdated today, the overall goals remain the same—to protect the brain and cells. At normal body temperature, the brain is not damaged for about five minutes after clinical death. With a decrease in body temperature, the brain is less dependent on oxygen and can be starved of oxygen for progressively longer periods of time. The body must be cooled, as protection of the brain is the prime consideration; this is truly the only irreplaceable organ. However, with the cooling, the doctor must prevent ice crystals from forming inside the cells. Water expands when it freezes, and since the human body is composed of more than 75 percent water, the cells would burst when the body is cooled below freezing. Special chemicals— such as glycerol with dimethyl sulfoxide (DMSO), which is injected into the bloodstream—absorb about 90 percent of the cells' water so that ice crystals form outside the cells rather than inside.

Also, the term *freeze* is somewhat of a misnomer. During perfusion, these chemicals cause the body to harden, or vitrify, like glass, not actually freeze, in order to minimize the damage to the body.

In the midst of this frenzied activity, Norman called. Dr. Bedford had changed his mind, saying that he was so old and decrepit he was not worth the effort or the money.

Professor Ettinger sent him a telegram and in one sentence changed Dr. Bedford's mind. Ettinger wrote, "Dr. Bedford, it is not a question of whether or not you are worth it, it is a question of whether such reanimation is possible—and if it is possible, then certainly you are worth it!"

When Dr. Bedford's perfusion became definite, I told Elaine. She was supportive and understanding, especially that night.

"That's really going to happen? You're really going to do this?" she asked. Elaine sounded cheery, with just a tinge of skepticism.

I nodded. I was grinning and floating and trying hard not to spin around the room. My little princess Susan felt the jubilation and danced around for me. I'd been slaving away for days, trying to coordinate all the manpower and the supplies; finally, with my family I allowed myself to indulge in some hard-won happiness.

My excitement was infectious. Elaine wrapped her arms around my neck and said, "I'm happy for you. I know you've wanted this." She leaned back, lifted my chin with her forefinger, and rocked her head back and forth, reading my eyes. "Wow, my husband is going to freeze the first man ever. Isn't that something?"

I grabbed her hands and said, "This'll change things for us. Are you ready?"

Elaine, ever the understanding wife and mother, just smiled and nodded.

I was anxious to meet Dr. Bedford; he was a courageous pioneer. A few days later I walked into his spartan room at the nursing home and saw that he was awake. Although he was obviously weak, his eyes blazed with a fire and awareness as he looked out an adjacent window.

I quietly walked to his bedside and introduced myself. After a pause, he looked at me, realizing I was the director of his impending suspension. With an ever-so-slight smile, he said in a hushed tone, "I have little hope of ever being reanimated, Mr. Nelson, but I believe in the future of cryonics. I hope my children or grandchildren will benefit from this inevitable medicine of the future." The sincerity in his eyes was clear and undeniable.

The next day, January 12, 1967, we substituted Dr. Renault Able for Dr. Bedford's attending physician.

Dr. Bedford was expected to live only a few more days, so we wanted to be ready when the time came. Robert and I had just picked up the necessary chemicals and were back in the office when Dr. Able called.

"I just pronounced him dead," he said.

I was caught off guard and didn't know what he was talking about at first. "Who?"

"Bedford! Who did you think?" He sounded more than a little anxious. "Did you procure the DMSO?"

"Shit!" I said, feeling disoriented. "I thought he had a couple days left."

"Patients tend not to wait for permission. Did you get the goddamned DMSO?"

"Yes. We just got back."

"Good. Please hurry. The scant amount of ice I have is starting to melt. You need to pick up more. He's on the heart compressor, but nothing else can happen until you arrive with those chemicals."

"We're on our way."

Dr. Able had witnessed Bedford's heart stop beating, pronounced him deceased, and then stepped aside. The perfusion team consisted of Dr. Brunol, Robert, and me in a treatment room at the nursing home. After we packed the patient in more ice, Dr. Brunol and Robert began injecting the biological antifreeze of 15 percent DMSO in Ringer's solution into Bedford's body. Heart compressions with the Westinghouse "Iron Heart" circulated the life-preserving liquid through his body. No blood was removed, as would become the practice in the future. By later standards, the two-hour perfusion process was crude. It was a primitive but glorious start. Robert commented in his 1969 book, *Suspended Animation,* that "the primitive equipment did not allow a precise measurement of DMSO penetration, but the perfusion appeared to be uniform."

We cooled down Dr. Bedford stepwise. The cryogenic cooling process began even before the perfusion, with Dr. Able surrounding the patient with ordinary water ice, at 32°F. When the perfusion was complete, Dr. Bedford was removed from the mountain of crushed ice and lifted from the operating table into a bed of much colder dry ice (-109°F) inside a wooden, polystyrene-lined container. He was then covered with more dry ice and transported to Robert's house. For permanent storage, Dr. Bedford would be immersed finally in liquid nitrogen, which is far colder yet, -320°F. At this final temperature, chemical and biological activity has practically ceased, and tissue will not decay for hundreds or even thousands of years.

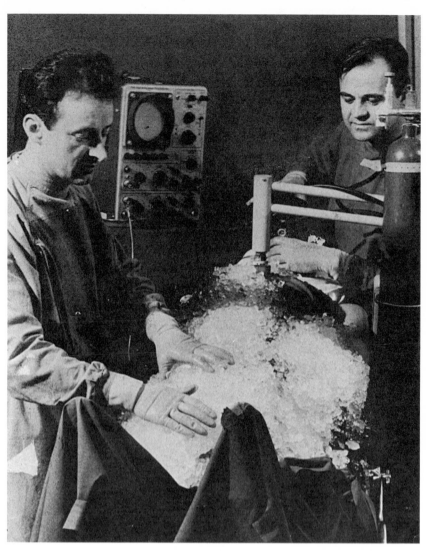

Freezing the first man: Dr. James Bedford

There was one rather bothersome detail I recall, fortunately not important for Dr. Bedford's preservation. Six hours later we moved the container to Robert's garage, a temporary storage location until Norman decided where to store his father's body. I opened the top of the container to see how the good doctor was faring with all this movement. When I removed the lid and checked him, I was concerned about a ten-pound block of dry ice, ten inches square by two inches thick; it was directly on top of his face, squishing the nose. Unfortunately, he was already frozen, so his nose would stay bent over for perhaps hundreds of years. I thought how dumb I was to not think about his nose and made a mental note for the next time. Other than that, he appeared to be in good condition. He was just a little bit dead, but he wasn't lost forever.

The next morning Robert's wife learned about the frozen body stored in her garage. Claudette screamed at her husband, calling him every derogatory name that her good breeding would allow. She gave him six hours or promised to call the police. Robert called me and ordered me to remove Dr. Bedford. I convinced my first-class hippie secretary, Sandra Stanley, and her easygoing husband, Shelby, to keep Dr. Bedford in their Topanga Canyon home. She smiled and shrugged, "What the hell; that's what friends are for."

I moved Dr. Bedford's body into the back of my Ford Ranchero pickup and then drove through the treacherous twisted roads of Topanga Canyon. I probably broke some laws—misdemeanor or felony, I couldn't be sure. However, a life was at stake.

About a week later, Norman wanted his father's body delivered to a mortuary service, which would transport Dr. Bedford to the Cryo-Care Equipment Co. in Phoenix, Arizona, for long-term placement in a cryogenic capsule.

Once again I drove Dr. Bedford in the back of my pickup the twenty miles through Topanga Canyon onto the Ventura Freeway to Balboa Park in the San Fernando Valley. With perhaps a hundred people milling about this enormous, plush green park and the sun perched high overhead, we transferred Dr. Bedford's huge, 350-pound dry-ice chest into the waiting black hearse. This was a first in world history—and no one noticed.

I waved him off as the hearse drove away. All the while the smoky vapors of dry ice billowed in the wind, declaring to the world, "Yes, I may be dead, but I'm just a little bit dead. And I will be back."

Headlines splashed the story of Dr. Bedford's freezing across the country and throughout the world. Professor Ettinger flew to California for a press conference with the CSC, and we gave at least thirty news media and television interviews and prepared for the lead story in an issue of *Life* magazine.

Professor Ettinger appeared on the *Johnny Carson Show* and most of the other top celebrity talk shows. Over time I appeared on *The Phil Donahue Show*, with Regis Philbin four times, and several others. While we were welcomed and treated with respect, the audiences seemed suspicious of greatly extended life and misconstrued cryonics as a replacement for an afterlife. Of course there can be an afterlife, be it heaven, nirvana, or the happy hunting ground, even if death is delayed.*

The scientific advisory council disintegrated. Robert told me that one of the researchers called after the freezing and said, "Don't mention our name; we want no part of this. It's over. Good-bye." They never phoned me. They wanted no association with the president of the body freezers.

Over the next twenty years, Dr. Bedford traveled a circuitous journey before he was donated to the Alcor Foundation in September 1987. They have since placed him in a state-of-the-art "Bigfoot" capsule that stands nine feet tall and holds several other patients, safely immersed in the -320°F chill of liquid nitrogen, making decay negligible. Because of Dr. Bedford's distinction as the first person cryogenically frozen, Alcor has pledged to maintain him until his reanimation, perhaps hundreds of years from today.

Immediately after Dr. Bedford's freezing, Dr. Able convinced Norman Bedford to create an independent partnership to conduct cryobiological research by informing him that the CSC was a bunch of amateurs. However, the partnership never was established. Young Bedford took custody

---

* Author's note: The complete story of Dr. Bedford's freezing and its immediate aftermath is described in my first book, *We Froze the First Man*, published in 1968.

of his father's body and had no further connection with CSC. He never paid for any of the services or material expenses extended by CSC in the freezing. The cost of this first freezing ultimately was covered by dues paid by CSC members, who nevertheless were honored to have participated.

What became of the three hundred thousand dollars left by Dr. Bedford to cover his expenses into perpetuity was a mystery to me for a long time. I now know that Norman used it in legal defense against other family members, who wanted to remove Dr. Bedford from suspension and acquire those funds for themselves. His relatives continued until the money was exhausted, which evaporated their incentive as well, so Dr. Bedford fortunately remained frozen. Norman deserves commendation for his dedication through all this, regardless of his financial standing with CSC.

I was delighted to learn that during the many years Dr. Bedford had been secretly moved from place to place, he had never thawed. Square-shaped ice cubes originally used to cool him were still intact. Therefore, we were confident that he stayed frozen during his entire suspension. This was enormously important to Alcor's decision to continue Dr. Bedford's suspension. Since then, he has remained safely immersed in the subzero chill of liquid nitrogen.

Dr. James Bedford was the first, but he was certainly not the last. Humankind continually strives to grow in the knowledge and revelations of our ever-changing universe. For us it might take more than a lifetime; but for the frozen patients, it requires only an instant.

CHAPTER 5

The Early Pioneers

AFTER THE CALLS FOR INTERVIEWS DECREASED and the furor died down, we entered a nebulous stage following Dr. Bedford's freezing. The scientific advisory board was gone, and while people were curious or titillated by the idea of cryonics, there were no patients and no significant donors. Being president of the CSC in search of donations made me feel like a serial dater—I was a man with an endless string of encounters, kissed at the end of the evening but never meeting someone willing to commit. The freezing of Dr. James Bedford had established our path: The CSC would continue finding patients who wanted to be frozen. We had brought the future to reality. The next time someone like Walt Disney called, we would be ready. In the aftermath, I was struggling to bring the CSC down the new direction I had forged.

That goal brought us together with a mortician, Joseph Klockgether, who saw that cryonics had the potential to grow into a worldwide phenomenon by changing the very definition of death. He discovered the CSC through a mortuary newsletter, which explained cryonics as an alternative form of interment. Joseph thought that cremating a person was a terrible waste and that cryonic suspension made more sense. He was exactly the type of mortician we needed.

After our initial conversations, Marshall Neel, our public relations director, and I went out to Rennaker Mortuary to meet with Joseph. He was in his early thirties and stood about five foot six, elegant and good mannered. I admired him because he wasn't concerned about what other people thought.

He greeted Marshall and me in the lobby of his mortuary and gestured for us to follow him to his office in the back. We walked past a chapel, three occupied visitation rooms, and a fully equipped embalming room, where he performed his typical duties in addition to autopsies. I looked around his office, found it practical but pleasant, and was intrigued by an old photograph of a horse-driven hearse over his desk; the driver wore a tall black hat and was dressed in formal attire.

Joseph told us that he was excited about cryonics and gladly would help with anything we asked. Since mortuaries tended to not return my phone calls, Joseph's willingness to help us was surprising.

Through cryonics, I was privileged to meet many passionate people with unconventional life stories. These kindred spirits became my friends, and we forged bonds far deeper than many I'd developed with my real family during my childhood.

In the car on the way to Santa Barbara, my good friend Sandra Stanley told me a little about the woman we were about to meet. "Marie's a leader in the feminist movement and involved in countless causes—the ACLU, the National Congress of American Indians, the Committee for a World Constitution, and the NAACP. She's interested in adding cryonics to the list." Sandra turned and looked at me. "Thank you so much for this trip. She's a mesmerizing woman, and I think she could do great things with us."

Back when Professor Ettinger was looking for someone to publish his book, he had sent out a hundred unsolicited copies of the manuscript to prominent scientists and activists listed in *Who's Who*. Marie Sweet had received one of these advance copies of *The Prospect of Immortality* and had been devoted to cryonics ever since.

As we drove up to her ancient brick house with a breathtaking ocean view, Marie came out the front door to greet us. "Hello there." She caught me in a full-on hug and said, "I've heard so much about all the amazing work you're doing, I'm just thrilled to meet you. I'd adopt you if I could.

Would you let me?" Marie gave me a sly smile and then moved on to a tighter, longer hug with Sandra.

Marie didn't fit my mental image of a feminist. She was an elderly lady who looked rather spent, but she offered to help any way she could. With her vast experience and sharp mind, she would prove invaluable.

While Sandra and Marie talked about their various foundations, I wandered into her husband's blacksmithing workshop, complete with a fiery kiln and giant anvil. Russ Le Croix Van Norden charmed me; he had a lilting walk and wore a black French beret slightly askew over his long

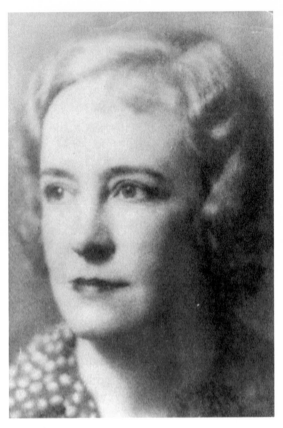

Marie Sweet

silvery hair. Although long past retirement age, he still built ornamental iron gates. When I mentioned Marie, a smile lit up his face. I could easily see how devoted he was to his wife and, by extension, to her causes. It touched my heart to see such tenderness in this elderly couple—the culmination of a lifelong love affair.

Both Marie and Russ joined our group and wanted to be frozen after their death. Marie worked miracles and convinced twenty scientists to write papers in biology, physiology, and space exploration and present them at the First National Cryonics Conference. Sadly, Marie never saw the presentations. On August 26, 1967, she traveled to Santa Monica and checked into a hotel for conference business. The next day she was scheduled to meet Sandra but never showed up. Sometime during the night, Marie died alone in the hotel room from heart failure.

We didn't find out for two days. During that time, the mortuary staff struggled to find her next of kin. Unbeknown to anyone, her husband was working in Salinas, and no other family could be found. Finally someone noticed the medical alert she wore on her wrist. The wristband identified her as a full body donor to the CSC, and the mortuary called me.

Abandoning all our conference duties, Sandra and I were frantically looking for Marie. When I learned the truth, I was spurred to quickly begin the freezing process. I tried contacting Joseph Klockgether, but he was out of town. He needed at least a day to get back to Santa Monica. Too much time had already elapsed, and she needed a perfusion soon to have even the slightest hope of being revived in the future.

I called Dr. Dante Brunol, who had performed the perfusion on Dr. James Bedford. He agreed to help, but he needed equipment and assistants. I then called Jeff Hicks, an apprentice at the California College of Mortuary Science. He told me he could bring equipment from the school and could assist. The next challenge was finding an operating room. The mortuary holding Marie's body wanted nothing to do with us, and we didn't want to waste time hunting for a willing mortuary.

I settled for an available operating room instead of a legal one. I called Jeff and said, "We have all the chemicals at our office in Westwood. Come here and we'll perform the perfusion on the desk."

Jeff and a fellow apprentice, Dennis Walker, picked up an embalming machine, ice, and all the other necessary equipment from the college. They took custody of Marie's body at the mortuary and then brought her to the CSC office.

We moved two big wooden desks side by side and covered them with green surgical sheets; then we removed Marie's body from her ice-filled body bag and placed her on the makeshift operating table. I laced up my surgical gown and triangulated myself between Marie, the office door, and the window overlooking the street below. Leaving the medical procedures to the doctor and the apprenticing morticians, I played the lookout, determined that they would finish the perfusion uninterrupted. Despite our precautions and protocols, I knew we couldn't legally perform the perfusion in this office building we shared with accountants and lawyers. Nervous and constantly playing with the ties on my surgical cap, I imagined the horrific headlines we'd see in tomorrow's newspaper if we were discovered.

I tried not to dwell on the wisdom of my rushed decisions over the past several hours, as this was neither the ideal location nor an ideal candidate for a perfusion. My heart dropped when I noticed that her abdomen was bloated and had turned a disturbing pale green.

Jeff noticed me staring at Marie's stomach instead the door. "It's the first part of the body to show decay after death—bacteria. We're lucky it hasn't been any longer. Once it starts, the decay process isn't pretty."

Her blood had pooled due to gravity, causing her back and sides to appear burgundy while her face was a ghostly white. I couldn't stomach the idea of that ultimately happening to me. Although natural, it seemed so unnecessary.

Jeff interrupted my thoughts. "I don't see any signs of insects. That's good."

I nodded and wished for an invisible mask of detachment to fall across my face. I wasn't optimistic about her future but wanted to continue the perfusion anyway. Ultimately, Marie's husband would decide whether to maintain her in an imperfect cryonic suspension or have her cremated. At least we could give him the option of suspension and a chance to fulfill Marie's wishes.

A cardiac pump machine was placed over her heart, forcing the blood to circulate and flow out of the body. Jeff started the embalming pump, which had a three-gallon reservoir of the perfusion liquid: mostly glycerol and dimethyl sulfoxide. These chemicals replaced the blood and would protect the patient's tissues when we cooled her body temperature below the freezing point of water. The formation of ice crystals would damage her cells and make it extremely difficult for future doctors to bring Marie back from her long ice nap.

Dr. Brunol picked up the scalpel, ready to make the first cut on Marie's carotid artery. For two hours he performed the perfusion while Jeff and Dennis kept her cooled. During the long procedure, I stole glances at the three men and felt in awe of their skill. Dr. Brunol's hands were deft and precise. This was only the second perfusion ever performed, and yet the apprentices expertly aided the doctor, anticipating his needs and having every tool ready as he called for it, although they'd never been taught this procedure at school.

When the operation was complete, they placed Marie in an aluminum casket liner and covered her with ice. They didn't completely fill the container until they brought her downstairs to the hearse.

We transported Marie to Joseph Klockgether's mortuary in Buena Park. Joseph was still out of town, but I grabbed the hidden key from underneath the flowerpot. We moved her into the empty garage and replaced the ice with dry ice to cool her to subzero temperature.

When it was all over, my hand lingered on the casket, feeling the cold aluminum. I now had the opportunity to mourn. "Goodbye, Marie," I said softly. "Dream not about today but of tomorrow."

Later, sinking into the front seat of the hearse, I dropped my head into my hands as the adrenaline drained away. Despite the roller coaster of that day's events, I just felt grateful that Marie rested on property legal to keep human remains. Marie Phelps-Sweet was the second person cryogenically frozen and the first woman. Allowing that thought to settle in my mind, it felt right. It seemed like a fitting coda for a woman who'd lived such an extraordinary life.

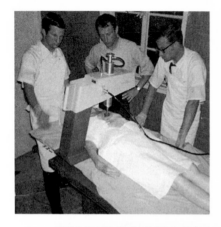
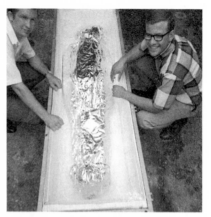
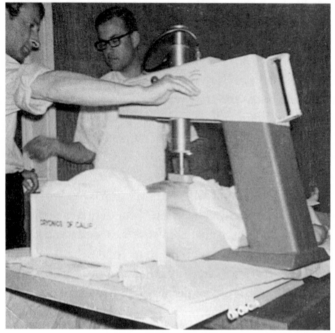

Dr. Dante Brunol and two apprentice morticians perform the perfusion on Marie Sweet in our Westwood offices, and then we place her inside the dry ice to keep her cold.

The media attention and drama surrounding the freezing of the first man, Dr. James Bedford, was absent this time. Her husband didn't even know she was dead yet.

Over the next few days, we built a wooden container for Marie from a large box originally used for shipping coffins. We insulated the inside and lid of the box with four inches of liquid polyurethane that solidified into a Styrofoam-like material. A second box was built to fit inside the larger, insulated one. Inside this second wooden box we placed Marie Sweet's body, along with several hundred pounds of dry ice. This configuration allowed Marie's body to be maintained at -109°F for a week before needing more dry ice.

I had the unenviable task of revealing to Russ that his wife was now frozen. A few days and countless phone calls later, I finally reached him. Although it was midmorning, he sounded groggy, as though he had just woken up.

I started tentatively. "Russ, have you heard the news?"

"Something about the conference? I got in late last night from that job up in Salinas. I think I have to slow it down—I'm too old to be working eighteen-hour days anymore. How's it going?"

My stomach sank. He didn't know, and I'd have to be the one to tell him.

"I'm dreadfully sorry to tell you this, but Marie died. The mortuary said it happened peacefully in her sleep." I continued to explain the details provided by the mortuary and all our efforts to locate him.

"She's gone? She died alone?" He went on like that—asking the same questions numerous times, alternating between the grief of a heartbroken husband and the practicality of dealing with the aftermath.

When the torrent of questions subsided, I broached the issue of the cryonics suspension.

"She's frozen? Oh, thank God. So she's not really gone." He exhaled deeply. "Thank you. Thank you. That meant so much to Marie. I'm so grateful to you."

Russ, undeterred by the amount of time between the death and freezing of Marie's body, asked that I maintain her in cryonic suspension.

Imperfect or not, barely feasible or not, Russ wanted this for Marie because she wanted it so much for herself. Near the end of the conversation, I finally broached the costs. "How much has Marie set aside for her suspension?"

A few moments of discouraging silence followed before he responded, "I'll need a few days to get back to you."

After hanging up, I began pricing capsules. Marie's freezing was, quite likely, never a viable suspension. She had been dead for several days, but we cryonicists are notorious optimists, and I had an unyielding faith that future scientific discoveries would render that two-day delay irrelevant. Marie's fate was now completely dependent on that faith. We had done our best. She had done so much for so many, and now she deserved for others to do for her.

With the freezing of Marie Sweet, the CSC now had its first frozen hero. Keeping Marie's body in perpetual suspension required money. The meager CSC budget depended on member dues, which weren't enough to cover day-to-day expenses. Knowing Marie, I was confident she had set aside at least the minimal amount necessary for her suspension. We needed to find a capsule, a permanent storage facility, and a liquid nitrogen provider. We were looking at at least ten thousand dollars to start, maybe more.

Russ showed up at my house a few days later. He pulled a wad of cash out of his pocket and laid it on the table.

"There's three hundred dollars, Bob," he said. "That's all the money we have."

Shocked, I stared at the meager pile of money. I had assumed Marie and Russ were financially secure. They lived in a gorgeous home overlooking the ocean, and he sold unique iron gates to wealthy people. Looking at Russ's forlorn expression, I knew he was telling me the truth.

I picked up the cash and rolled the bills around in my hand. "Is that all?" I asked. Three hundred dollars would pay for only a month of dry ice.

"That's it," he said. "We've mostly been living on our Social Security. I know it's not enough to keep her in suspension. Please do whatever you can."

How could I say no? I dropped the money back on the table, and it landed next to a family photo of Elaine and me. I remembered that Russ cherished Marie the way I loved my wife. I would fight for Marie. "I'll keep her in temporary storage as long as possible. Perhaps with some publicity generated by the suspension, and a little arm-twisting within the cryonics community, enough money could be raised."

Russ Van Norden, Russ Stanley, and I set out to find donations for Marie Sweet's suspension. I wrote Professor Ettinger, asking if he could raise money from the membership of the Cryonics Society of Michigan. He replied with a personal check for one hundred dollars to help Marie. While hope, passion, and faith were plentiful within the cryonics community, cash always seemed to be a scarce commodity. His donation was generous and touching. He wrote, "I'll see what can be done locally, but I'm doubtful we can raise any substantial sum."

In Russ's impassioned plea to the cryonics community and his wife's numerous organizations, he gave voice to the motivations and dreams of all our members:

Tears dim my eyes and anguish wrenches at my heart as I recall with crystal clarity my wife's many crusades for the peaceful communication of mankind. I am humbled that I have done so little in comparison. As many of you now know, she lies carefully but critically suspended, no different in essence than when you knew her yesteryear. If she has touched your cause and organization, then you may have felt her contribution and feel moved to give your kind aid.

Perhaps it could be said of her that she had everything except money, for the great and near great counted her as a friend. From East to West and even abroad, she helped to weave the fabric of some good Cause for the benefit and enlightenment of mankind.

I touched her hair and kissed her now cold lips in a farewell for what may well be only a few short years. Swiftly developing science may remove her from her minus-zero suspended animation and return her here among us—her enthusiasm undimmed.

If you would dare believe this is possible, the need is now for funds for cryogenic care until the final sealing of her enclosing capsule for the long wait of months or years ahead. Hers was an ideal passing, and traditional fears only hover at the outer edge of my consciousness. For I believe in steadfast earnestness that she will come back to us.

Russ Le Croix Van Norden

His letter received a torrent of sympathy mail and emotional support, but little money. We contemplated our other options, but none of our efforts proved successful.

Joseph Klockgether agreed to keep Marie Sweet in his unused garage on his mortuary grounds until we could obtain a capsule and a permanent storage facility. Those twin tasks were far more arduous than I had envisioned. First there was the dry ice, which had to be replenished every week and cost ninety dollars. Often there weren't enough funds in the CSC bank account to cover the weekly replenishment, and I had to withdraw the money from my personal account. Sometimes I had to choose between paying my mortgage and paying for dry ice. And with each dollar spent on dry ice, we were a dollar further away from a permanent solution.

Thus began my weekly ritual of transporting the dry ice across Los Angeles to Joseph's mortuary, which I would perform for the next two years. I usually left around ten or eleven o'clock in the morning to avoid the worst of the traffic during my fifty-mile trek on the Ventura Freeway between my home in Woodland Hills and the Rennaker Mortuary in Buena Park. The ninety-minute trip could extend to three hours, the dry ice slowly subliming in my backseat. The cold permeated the seats and froze the upholstery on my Porsche Speedster; eventually the leather seats looked like black prunes.

One Saturday I was sitting in traffic, watching the dry ice slowly disappear in my rearview mirror. I wanted action, and yet all I seemed to be doing was sitting, waiting, and accomplishing nothing more than my friends lying in stasis. In an effort to move, to do *something*, I pulled my car over to the freeway shoulder and buried my face in my hands. "Am

I crazy?" I said aloud. "What the hell am I doing? This is madness." My breathing grew shallow and fast as I fought the temptation to take the dry ice from the backseat and shuck it off the overpass. It would be an ending.

I balled my hands into fists so tight that my nails cut into the fleshy part of my palms and tried to calm myself. I repeated memorable lines from Professor Ettinger's book, from his appearances, and from our conversations. I made a mental checklist of all the supporting documentation about cryonics and convinced myself again of its logic. I looked out the window and marveled at a weed growing from the narrowest imaginable crack in the dry asphalt. "Yes, this is logical," I resolved. "But it's also crazy. Life is crazy. And life always finds a way." I shrugged, resigned once again to my fate of these weekly sojourns of dry-ice replenishment and feeling confident that these were messy but necessary steps toward our goal of future reanimation.

At the mortuary I pulled up to the garage and unloaded the dry ice. Marie's container was kept below a wide shelf on rollers so it could be pulled out. I removed the lid and placed the dry ice around her sides, which gave me the opportunity to visually inspect her condition every week. I wanted to make sure she was still solidly frozen and she didn't have skin burns from the dry ice. Her face and features looked identical to when we had our last conversation. There was no deterioration or alteration; not even her blue pantsuit seemed changed. Once satisfied, I covered her with the remaining dry ice, starting with her face and then working down to her feet. Finally I replaced the lid and rolled her container back into place. The procedure usually took about forty-five minutes.

I dreaded trying to find Joseph at the mortuary. I wandered around the facility calling for him, but I inevitably located him in the embalming room. Many times I'd gone there and found Joseph standing over a body on the operating table. In those moments, the macabre reality of death came upon me. Sometimes the corpse was cut open, the intestines lying on the table.

I hoped that with all my efforts, embalming would be reduced. That practice seemed horrendously wasteful—it only temporarily preserved the appearance of life, while we wanted to preserve life itself.

When remembering the history of the cryonics movement in which I was privileged to participate, I could not forget a frail, tiny lady named Helen Kline—the woman who hosted our first California cryonics meetings. While in the final stages of lung cancer, Helen read *The Prospect of Immortality*. She was a motivating force from the beginning. Although only in her mid- to late fifties, she was quite frail. During the meetings in her home, she often excused herself with her frequent coughing fits.

One time she asked me to accompany her to the grocery store. When we arrived at the market, she kept her arm hooked in mine and paraded around the store instead of actually shopping. I noticed all her friends staring and whispering about me. I realized I wasn't providing assistance but rather arm candy. Playing the role she wanted, I strutted with her, hoping to provide the most memorable impression on behalf of this indomitable lady.

On May 14, 1968, I received a call from her sister at Los Angeles General Hospital. "I'm Maryann, Helen's sister. She asked me to phone you several days ago, and I'm sorry it took me so long. She's in a coma now, and her doctors say her condition is deteriorating fast."

"Thanks so much for calling," I replied. As I had learned too well with Marie Sweet, advance knowledge and preparation were vital. "Are you aware that Helen is a major figure in cryonics? She has signed all the necessary documents to have her body frozen at death."

"I am aware of the legal papers."

Her curt tone worried me, so I rushed to Helen's bedside.

When I arrived at the hospital, I could see Helen was near the end. Her skin was a shocking blue-gray, and she was flanked by countless machines. Nurses hurried in and out of the room to check her monitors. Maryann was holding Helen's hand; she was about sixty, with a heap of gray hair stacked high on her head.

Since I wasn't sure if Helen could hear us, I asked Maryann to follow me into the hallway. "Has your sister made any financial arrangements for cryonics suspension?"

She held up her hand. "There's no need to discuss this. I have no money, and neither does Helen. While you were on your way here, she regained consciousness and told me she changed her mind and does not want her body frozen. She wants to be cremated."

Her statement ignited a slow burn in my gut. "Really?" I replied. "Are you telling me that very coincidentally, as I was rushing down here to make arrangements to place her in suspended animation, she miraculously came out of a coma just long enough to tell you that she had changed her mind and wanted to be cremated, then conveniently went back into her coma?"

She sheepishly answered, "Well, yes."

I did not want to further upset the woman, but I couldn't allow her to interfere with Helen's wishes. Firmly yet gently I told her, "I think it would be wise for you to back off, unless you want a lawsuit you couldn't possibly win."

I was bluffing. Cryonics was controversial, and a good outcome wasn't guaranteed, regardless of Helen's wishes. Besides, once Helen was declared clinically dead, any legal delay would be devastating to a successful perfusion.

Fortunately, Maryann backed down; she didn't want a fight any more than I did.

I quickly began preparations for Helen's perfusion at the moment she was declared dead. I told the hospital staff that the CSC was a cryobiological research organization, Helen was a medical donor, and she needed to be covered in ice so that we could accept her donation. To my relief, they cooperated. When Joseph Klockgether arrived at the hospital to retrieve Helen's body, she was already packed in ice and waiting at the loading dock.

Joseph brought her to his mortuary and performed the perfusion. He then placed Helen in the temporary storage container with Marie Sweet and covered her with dry ice. The entire process from death to temporary storage took about seven hours. Thanks to the cooperation from the hospital and Joe's swift action, Helen Kline was frozen under the best conditions.

I thought of a movie I had seen recently, *Planet of the Apes.* While Charlton Heston was portraying a suspended NASA astronaut hurtling toward a distant planet, mimicking what we hoped to accomplish, I was busy freezing Helen Kline and struggling to make this science-fiction notion into reality.

The CSC members unanimously agreed that we should try to give Helen a chance at long-term suspension. We had our second frozen hero, but we had yet to take on our first paying patient.

When remembering the early history of cryonics, it is impossible to ignore this frail little woman. While in the final stages of lung cancer, Helen overcame her pain and suffering and found the strength to organize the first California cryonics meeting. I am forever indebted to her.

— ∼ —

I met Russ Stanley at that first meeting of California cryonicists in Helen's home. He was a tall, slender older-looking gentleman with an obnoxious Cheshire cat grin, but quite athletic. He swam laps in his aboveground pool every day, even on the coldest winter morning.

Every day for the next two years, he called and talked to me for hours if I couldn't find a way to escape. It seemed he ate, drank, and slept cryonics. If there was anything about cryonics going on, anywhere in the country, he knew about it.

He had accumulated every newsletter and article ever published on cryonics, enough to stuff a full-size file cabinet. His genuine enthusiasm was infectious, and he often provided great little pearls of new information.

On September 6, 1968, I was in San Francisco organizing a new cryonics society. During the meeting, Paul Porcasi, the CSC secretary, phoned me that Russ had suffered a heart attack and been taken to the Santa Fe Medical Center in Los Angeles, where he had been pronounced dead.

The hospital staff ignored the documentation Russ carried on him, which gave specific instructions to cool his body with ice at the moment of his death and to contact the CSC immediately. Instead they contacted

Rosario, a man I had met at Russ's house, who was listed as next of kin. Rosario thought cryonics was ridiculous, but he respected Russ's wishes and fulfilled them the best he could.

Paul was a nervous wreck. The hospital refused to cool Russ's body without consent from the attending physician—an infuriating stance, because brain damage began shortly after death. Rapid cooling slowed the deterioration and, in theory, preserved the memory of the patient. I adored Russ and wanted to give him the best chance for a full recovery.

I used my most authoritative tone, hoping to spur him into action: "Paul, contact Joseph Klockgether and ask him to meet you at the hospital. The hospital needs to release his body to Joseph. Also, bring along all Russ's donation papers—they're on file in my office."

"Should I also bring the CSC's articles of incorporation?" he asked.

I felt powerless so far from Los Angeles. I replied, "Bring them, but don't go flashing them around."

Hospitals at that time were skittish of freezing bodies for later reanimation, but they were receptive to anatomical donations for medical research. If he approached the staff as a research organization, he had a better chance of receiving their assistance.

They finally cooperated. Joseph took possession of Russ's body, covered him with ice, and brought him to the mortuary. After the perfusion, his body was placed alongside Marie Sweet and Helen Kline. A total of six hours had elapsed between the time of Russ's death and the start of his perfusion. Like Marie's perfusion, the intervening time made this an imperfect operation. If Russ ever opened his eyes, he would likely have memory loss, but his suspension was still considered viable.

The day I returned from San Francisco, I contacted Rosario Coco. Russ had made Rosario executor of his estate, and I was anxious to learn the financial arrangements for his suspension. I knew Russ had impeccable records and documentation; no individual was more prepared for cryonic suspension. However, there was still the enormously important matter of financial arrangements.

Russ had told me he had a substantial bank balance. Although it didn't cost more to keep him in temporary storage with Marie and Helen, we couldn't sustain them forever—we desperately needed funding for a permanent storage facility. Russ knew our needs, knew our limitations, and surely had left sufficient funds to finally accomplish the task.

Russ had described Rosario as his "sweetheart from way back." That was no real surprise to me—I had suspected Russ was gay when he introduced me to Rosario at the first meeting. To me the man looked like an owl. Rosario had big rings around his eyes and a tiny beak of a nose. He was small, with wavy gray hair and a curt personality. I knew that Russ had trusted this man and thought the world of him.

In his will, Russ bequeathed ten thousand dollars to the CSC, payable in two five-thousand-dollar installments. I was stunned, as I had anticipated at least double that amount to accomplish Russ's suspension and perpetual storage. I delicately grilled his friend about the funds to pay for Russ's suspension. He brusquely retorted, "That's all I know."

Obviously Rosario wanted to dismiss us, but he was executor, and I wasn't going to make it easy for him. I asked, "Was this a donation to the CSC, or were we expected to freeze and store him perpetually for that amount?"

He said, "I have no idea," then abruptly ended the conversation with "Good-bye."

I stared at the telephone receiver until my backside begged me to get out of the stiff wooden office chair. Once again I found myself in the peculiar position of placing another patient in temporary storage when I knew the CSC couldn't provide perpetual maintenance. Russ's total purpose in his later life, at least during the years I knew him, was supporting the research of cryonics science. I was surprised to learn that one of the most fanatical and wealthy cryonics advocates had left only ten thousand dollars for his suspension. I knew Rosario was an honest man—Russ must've underestimated the necessary funds. I would have to invest the money he did provide wisely. It had to stretch a long way.

CHAPTER 6

The Vault

CSC's MEMBERSHIP HAD GROWN TO NEARLY ONE HUNDRED. Anticipating a deluge of cryonics requests, we set up a for-profit corporation to design, develop, and provide cryogenic hardware equipment for CSC's future needs. Marshall Neel was the president of this company, Cryonic Interment, since he had been our business brain. He was a refreshing counterweight that kept me—the passionate, optimistic dreamer—grounded. I loved his objectivity and realism; he'd often say "Change wives, change problems."

Our plan was to have CSC contract with CI to perform perfusions and store suspended members. Despite our current meager funds, we felt assured about the future of cryonics. With that optimism and Russ Stanley's donation, we wanted a permanent storage facility.

Finding and setting up the proposed facility was far more difficult than I had imagined. Since the law limited storage of bodies at a mortuary to less than six months, the city of Buena Park wanted Marie, Helen, and Russ out of the Rennaker Mortuary. The health department had extended the deadline for us several times but was getting impatient. Joseph Klockgether had pleaded with me, "Build your vault, Bob, and get your people out of here." If we couldn't store bodies at Joseph's mortuary, how could we get past regulations for storing them at our own facility?

The answer turned out to be surprisingly simple and practical. We could build an underground vault in a cemetery. There we would be immune from the local laws of legal disposition of our frozen patients. I also had to face the grim possibility of failure, since the technology was still experimental. With the patients already in a cemetery, they would be considered legally interred. Should the cryonics program dissolve, they could remain in the vault unless family members decided otherwise.

It sounded so uncomplicated, but finding a willing cemetery wasn't easy. Joseph used his contacts, but the answer we kept hearing was "No, there's no precedent for such interments."

Of course I knew the real reason for the rejections. Cemetery directors didn't mind dealing with dead people—just as long as they stayed dead. Future reanimation was all too new and strange for them to accept. After months of abysmal luck, a beam of Southern California sun finally permeated through.

My mother-in-law had recently purchased two plots at the Oakwood Memorial Park Cemetery in Chatsworth, a suburb of Los Angeles. It was a beautiful place with rolling hills, surrounded by picturesque mountains—an ideal place to be dead, I suppose. I found their number in the Yellow Pages and called the office. I explained that CSC was a nonprofit cryobiological research organization and that we were looking for a place to store medical remains for research. I received an appointment to see the owner, Frank Enderle, immediately.

He was a cordial gentleman and listened politely. As soon as I mentioned cryonics, he leaned back in his chair and knew exactly what I wanted. To my surprise, he told me he would think about it. His brother was on the California State Cemetery Board, and he wanted his brother's legal advice before making a decision.

Frank wasn't bothered by the idea of hosting a cryonics facility as long as the cemetery had no liability. Once he received the go-ahead from his brother, he responded to me, insisting that the underground facility be constructed using the rigorous mausoleum code.

On my third visit, Frank drove me through the cemetery to choose a location. Just two hundred feet beyond the main offices, I found the perfect spot. The ground was level and situated close to the road, making it easily accessible to liquid-nitrogen delivery trucks. I didn't really expect Frank to agree, but he once again surprised me, and I successfully obtained that location.

Although Frank was not interested in cryonics, he was intrigued by its novelty. While I wrote out the check for the large plot, his general manager, a tall lanky man named Chuck, walked into the office.

Frank asked him, "Do you have any objections to having the cryonics vault on cemetery grounds?"

My heart was in my mouth; I feared he might say something to obstruct us.

A thoughtful look flashed across Chuck's face. "I do have one concern. How many frozen people could be in that vault?"

I put on my most trustworthy, concerned expression and answered, "At the very most—twenty."

After a long pause, he looked me straight in the eye. "What are you going to do if they wake up and start fucking and fighting down there?"

My serious face broke into a huge grin. It was good to know that they had a sense of humor. They certainly needed it in later years.

I contracted a company to build the vault. It was constructed of steel rebar and cement, much like a swimming pool, with interior dimensions of twelve by eighteen feet. A door was built into the steel roof, which slid horizontally on rollers. A ladder led from the door at grass level to the bottom. Meanwhile, we had to find a capsule for our frozen heroes to rest in long-term suspension—but the capsules weren't cheap.

At this point, between the plot of land and the construction of the still-unfinished vault, CSC had spent close to seven thousand dollars of Russ's ten-thousand-dollar donation.

We lucked into finding a tank that could hold thirty patients at an industrial liquidation yard in Los Angeles. Only slight modifications were necessary, since it had all the instrumentation to monitor the core temperature and liquid nitrogen boil-off.

The top of the massive capsule had a sealed lid, which allowed access to the patients. The five-thousand-dollar price tag was a bargain; the original purchase invoice showed the capsule had cost nearly $150,000. There were, however, some serious downsides. First, the capsule was too large to fit in the plot we had already purchased, and we didn't have the money to build a new, larger vault. Second, we'd need a lot of liquid nitrogen to fill its cavernous interior, as well as the money to maintain it. Marshall and I figured five or six paying suspensions would finance the capsule, but we had an immediate need for our current cases.

In the end we banked on our optimism and took a leap of faith with the big capsule. CSC had around twenty-five-hundred dollars left in its bank account, and I arranged for a loan to pay the rest. Frank allowed us to store the capsule in the cemetery's heavy-equipment yard until we found it a permanent home and Cryonic Interment could begin using it. We were excited about the future. Soon we would have the paying suspensions to operate our new, state-of-the-art facility.

I was selling cryonics and our new facility to the public, traveling the country, giving presentations, and talking about CSC's new capabilities. After interviews on several national television and radio talk shows, I was flying high and feeling golden. A guy like me from my background, on radio and television, was seen as an expert?

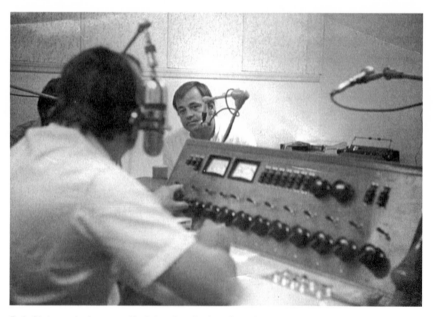

Bob Nelson during a radio interview in Los Angeles

My wife was amused by the media attention but embarrassed by its bizarreness. She focused on the children and tried filling the void created by my long hours away from home. The kids enjoyed seeing their dad interviewed on TV at first, but it soon became mundane. One time I sat down to watch the replay of an interview with *Channel 5 News;* however, my daughter Lori was already watching a program and didn't care to switch the channel to see her dad.

I always felt confident that with all the exposure, we were just one phone call, one more TV appearance, one interview, just one more day away from financial solvency. I hated feeling so focused on cash though. I had such big goals—we were fighting for the future of humanity—and yet here I was in this position of going after the money.

Robert Prehoda and Dr. Brunol still came to dinners and gave talks, but since there was no money, they just gradually faded away. In our newsletter we boasted of the world's first cryotorium—a proclamation I later regretted, because my detractors claimed I had overstated our accomplishments. But we were desperate for paying suspensions, and I thought a little exaggeration was justified. Hundreds of letters and phone

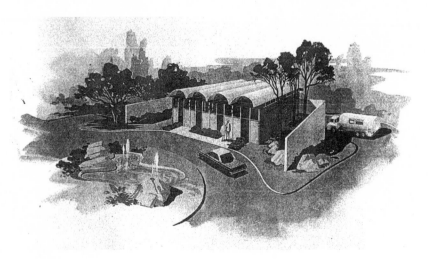

Artist conception of future CSC cryonics facility

calls were pouring into CSC, and people were signing up. Still, there were no new patients, and the expenses just continued to mount. I didn't know how much longer I could hang on, but I couldn't think about failure. Somehow, I hoped we could save our frozen heroes.

In late 1968 we encountered another turn of fortune. Louis Nisco had been in cryonic suspension at Cryo-Care Equipment Corporation in Phoenix, Arizona, for a year. His daughter, Marie Brown, was desperate. She could no longer afford the monthly storage and liquid-nitrogen maintenance payments, and Ed Hope, who owned the company, was threatening to terminate the suspension. Marie had purchased her father's capsule from Ed for forty-eight hundred dollars. She still owed fifteen hundred dollars and was making monthly payments along with storage and liquid nitrogen fees. She couldn't keep up with the payments and wanted my help. I called Ed Hope to get his side of the story. Ed was a businessman, pure and simple. His main line of work was manufacturing wigs, but when he saw an opportunity to make money, he added on the business of cryonics capsules.

Ed and I appeared together once on the *Louis Lomax* television show. That was during the summer of 1966, and it was my first-ever TV appearance. The producer of the show asked if I could bring a visual demonstration. I told him I had just returned from a visit to Ed's Cryo-Care facility in Phoenix and would ask him if he could bring a capsule to the show. I didn't need to ask Ed twice. The *Louis Lomax* show was nationally syndicated, and it meant big-time sales potential to Ed. He showed up at my house two days before the show, pulling a trailer with CRYO-CARE and HUMAN SUSPENDED ANIMATION EQUIPMENT plastered all over it. My wife was mortified about what the neighbors thought.

Three minutes before the show, Ed was still in his dressing room. I went in and asked what was keeping him. He was frantic. He couldn't find his toupee and refused to go onstage without it. At that moment Lomax grabbed me and said we had only one minute left—forget about Ed. He got me onto the soundstage just in time. I was a nervous wreck; it felt like I had eaten a cotton ball sandwich for lunch. Lomax introduced me to the live audience as "the guy who could get you frozen and bring you back."

My secretary told me afterwards that I looked like someone desperately in need of a bathroom. I managed to parrot some of the things I'd heard Professor Ettinger say about cryonics, and our forty-five-minute segment stretched to an hour and fifteen minutes. An audience member asked if people should wear something warm for their suspension, which loosened me up. Eventually Ed came out, wig neatly arranged on his melon, and demonstrated his capsule. He managed to mention his phone number, just in case someone wanted to buy one.

Ed Hope was ruthless; if he couldn't make a buck, then he wouldn't waste his time. When I asked him about Marie's situation, he told me, "If that capsule isn't out of here in two weeks, I'm going to kick the fucking thing into the street. Is there any part of that you don't understand?"

I understood all right—Ed meant exactly what he said. I called Marie, and she was badly shaken and needed an immediate resolution. I saw an opportunity: I badly needed a capsule, since the big one couldn't be used yet, and she needed someone to store her father at a price she could afford. I offered to pay the remaining balance she owed on the capsule and to take charge of her father's suspension. In return, I asked that she donate her father and the capsule to CSC and continue making payments of $150 per month to cover the costs of storage and liquid nitrogen. I told her of our plans to eventually get our large capsule ready and that we would transfer her father to the capsule at that time. She gratefully accepted.

I mentioned there might be some shuffling of bodies before we got our large capsule functioning, but I didn't provide specifics. In truth, I wanted to open her father's capsule and place Marie Sweet, Helen Kline, and Russ Stanley in there with him. I wasn't completely honest with her, but I figured that since she was donating the capsule to CSC, we could do what we wanted—and we had a real need. I reasoned that if they were reanimated, it would be more fun to be part of a group of survivors rather than be a lonely, solitary product of an experiment. Nevertheless, of all my dealings in cryonics, this omission bothered my conscience the most.

Marshall Neel drew up the papers that donated Louis Nisco's body to CSC under the Uniform Anatomical Gift Act, along with the capsule, and Marie signed them. I called Ed and informed him that I would drive to Arizona to retrieve the Nisco capsule the next day.

He asked, "Did she give you any money for me?"

When I responded no, he said, "Come and get the fucking thing before I do something I'll be sorry for."

Ed was paying for the liquid nitrogen himself, something he detested. He confided, "I'm getting out of this fucking business. It's all a bunch of crazy people and crazy problems."

I'd never met anyone so contradictory with his name—nothing about him made me think of hope—*Ed Avarice* would have been far more appropriate. I told him the CSC was prepared to give him the fifteen hundred dollars owed by Marie upon picking up the capsule. Suddenly we became very popular with Ed.

I rented a heavy-duty truck and trailer and set off to pick up the capsule. A close friend, Fred Martin, joined me for the ride. Fred was an insurance wizard who was developing a plan to provide coverage for suspension costs. We arrived at Cryo-Care on a Saturday morning, and Ed treated us to breakfast at his favorite hangout. Mouth agape, I watched him devour a huge stack of blueberry pancakes along with three eggs, sausage, bacon, two huge scoops of vanilla ice cream, milk, and countless cups of coffee. Yes, Ed Hope was a big man. For me he was a reinterpretation of Scrooge's comment to Jacob Marley: "There's more of gravy than of grave about you."

We started back to California that same morning. On the way, outside some little Arizona town, we ran out of fuel thanks to a faulty gas gauge on the rental truck. I was debating my options when I saw a highway patrolman in my rearview mirror. *Great!* I looked over at Fred and raised my eyebrows, trying to signal to him to play it cool.

The officer pulled up alongside my window. "What's the problem?"

Thinking of our unusual cargo, I tried to act nonchalant; but I was sweating from the heat. "I'm not sure. It feels like we ran out of gas, but the gauge shows we've got a third of a tank."

The policeman perched his sunglasses in his hair, rolled up his sleeves, and lifted the hood of the truck. After a few minutes of tinkering, he confirmed we were out of gas. I just sat there, sticking to the fake leather seat and dreading that he'd ask me to step out of the truck to show him what I was hauling in the trailer. Instead he pulled out a clear plastic hose from his trunk and hooked it up to a special spot on his carburetor. Out rushed gas directly into my tank, three gallons free of charge, courtesy of rinky-dink Arizona. As we drove off, I asked our cargo, Louis Nisco, to say good-bye to the officer.

Back at Joseph's mortuary, our luck hadn't changed. Marie broke all our agreements and never gave the CSC the monthly payments she promised. Not long after we transferred the capsule to the mortuary, she sent me a handwritten note that she was leaving the fate of her father to me and whatever happened was in CSC's hands. We needed the income badly, but in a way I was elated. Her letter freed me from worry over her possibly discovering I had used the capsule for several people, as well as any liability. Or so I thought. I didn't hear from Marie again until years later, under far different circumstances.

—◆—

I felt the curious warmth of hope mingled with apprehension. However, I should have refused Ed Hope's offer to take ownership of the capsule and keep its patient at -320°F for the next several hundred years. This proto-type leaked badly and required a vacuum pump continuously to maintain a half-decent vacuum between the outer wall and inner chamber. The liquid nitrogen needed replacing every week instead of just once a month, but the allure of placing our four patients into this single capsule was far too thrilling to turn down. Hauling dry ice a hundred miles every week for two years was a nightmare of labor and expense, especially since only Russ had left any money to pay for this journey.

On a cold morning in March 1969, I met Joseph Klockgether in his mortuary garage with a huge agenda for the day. We were opening the Louis Nisco capsule and placing the other three patients inside. I couldn't sleep the night before; I was too worried about this daunting task. If not sealed perfectly, we risked making an already leaky, decrepit capsule even worse.

These patients—Marie, Helen, and Russ—had been our friends and our kindred spirits in the cryonics movement. This was the first time in history anyone had attempted such lifesaving efforts; we respected this maiden voyage and did everything possible to honor them. It was my fervent hope this capsule would save these people who were gambling on future technology.

Ray Fields, a welding expert, had called me to offer his services. After examining his credentials and prior work, I agreed. He was eager to help, arriving at the mortuary garage before I did. We needed three hours to open the capsule, as the cut had to be perfect so that it could be welded back exactly as before and sealed correctly. During this time, Marie, Helen, and Russ remained in their temporary storage container with dry ice. New to our mission, Ray stared in awe at their perfectly preserved bodies.

Ray hovered over the capsule with his diamond saw, preparing to make the first cut. His face was scrunched up, looking concerned. "Is he going to be okay?" he asked, gesturing to the now-drained capsule with Louis Nisco still inside.

I was pouring some coffee for Joseph and me from the percolator. "Don't worry; a body at liquid-nitrogen temperature doesn't thaw in a few hours, so we have plenty of time. Just think about Thanksgiving turkey. Every year, my wife Elaine leaves a fifteen-pounder on our kitchen counter overnight to thaw. In the morning, its center is usually still frozen."

Ray nodded, understanding, his attention focused on the sliver-thin cut progressing along the stainless-steel capsule.

I felt a little odd talking turkey, but I had needed to reach for strange analogies to explain cryonics principles over the years. "Now imagine that same bird weighed 120 pounds and was frozen at 320 degrees below zero; that turkey would be frozen solid for days. Louis is quite safe—as long as we don't spend a week trying to get this perfect."

We began by releasing the vacuum between the two chambers. A cryogenic capsule is a giant thermos bottle with a vacuum drawn between the inner and outer cylinders. I explained to Ray that vacuum was the best possible insulation to maintain the four-hundred-degree temperature difference between the inner capsule and the Southern California weather. "It's interesting that humans can't survive in a vacuum or in liquid nitrogen, but both are necessary ingredients to preserve these lives."

After Ray cut open the capsule and we spent four exhaustive hours positioning our friends, we had all four patients inside the rickety Nisco capsule. After the capsule was bolted and sealed, we connected the vacuum pump, recharged it with liquid nitrogen, and said a little prayer.

After checking the capsule every day for two weeks, I knew we were in terrible trouble. The vessel was worse than before. Even with the vacuum pump running continuously, the liquid nitrogen was disappearing quickly; I knew I couldn't maintain the expense for very long. I felt frustrated and abandoned. I tried hard to not snap at the people helping me, especially Joseph and my wife Elaine.

We intended to keep the capsule at the mortuary until the vault was completed, but the health department was pressuring Joseph to relocate the frozen bodies. In May 1970 we moved the capsule to the Oakwood Memorial Park Cemetery in Chatsworth. Instead of placing the capsule into the vault, which had no electricity or ventilation, we placed it in the heavy equipment yard alongside the huge thirty-man capsule. If that were operational, it would solve all our problems, but instead it sat empty, silently mocking me. Frank Enderle gave me almost free rein at the cemetery to accomplish a goal that was becoming harder and harder to achieve. But failure was not an option; I just had to keep pushing forward.

Sometimes opportunities ride in on the wind, and sometimes they tap your shoulder. Months passed while the vault remained unfinished. Then late in the year, I befriended a gentleman named Frank Farrell. Frank was an anomaly, a defiant deviation from the standard order of human beings—he was exactly the opposite of what he appeared to be.

I was at a Santa Monica engineering office, trying to build a steel frame for the convertible top of my 1952 Porsche. Mine had been stolen while the Speedster was parked in downtown Westwood, and I was looking for someone who could fabricate this part for me. The frame had been unavailable from the Porsche dealer for more than ten years, and I had spent a year to find it.

I had just been told the usual "no way" by some so-called expert when Frank, who had been standing behind me, introduced himself. He looked as though he had just climbed out of a Dumpster. His clothes were a mess and likely had never seen an iron. Frank was about six feet tall, had poor posture, and could not have weighed an ounce over 120 pounds—a hunched human scarecrow. He had an enormous Adam's apple, and his top front teeth protruded from his smile.

He announced that he could build me the part if he could copy an original. I was doubtful at first, but as we talked I could see this was no hobo. We had lunch and conversed for hours. Frank had no interest in the material trappings of life. He had no home or automobile. He lived intermittently with each of his three daughters. He made good money as an engineer and supported all three of his daughters but owned nothing of his own, except for a paper shopping bag he toted around in his filthy hands. Technical expertise aside, I wondered how his employer tolerated his appearance.

For one hundred dollars, Frank fabricated a perfect copy of the frame I needed. He installed it on my vehicle with a special bolt system so that no one could steal it again.

The man was brilliant. Over the course of a half-dozen years, Frank proved himself to be a magician in mangy dog clothing. He helped build the cryonics vault and skillfully maintained the rickety cryogenic capsules, along with our six testy high-vacuum pumps. He averted disaster countless times.

Frank refused to budge about his hygiene though. Sometimes I cringed, but I would put an invisible clothespin over my nose and remember the olfactory fortitude I had developed when I was a homeless teenager. Remembering those days, I couldn't fathom how someone would choose to live with that stink. Nevertheless, he was a gift from heaven, a lovable friend who knew everything about everything.

He fixed each problem one by one. He brought in an aqualung and fans to improve air circulation. Also, I was paranoid about security. We didn't want anyone knowing about the vault, entering the vault, or taking pictures of the vault, so Frank installed a high-tech lock that required a key turned a specific way or an alarm would sound.

I had recently seen *2001: A Space Odyssey*, which had these mysterious black monoliths that were endowed with mystical powers of creation. Frank showed me plans for our vault cover, about ten feet long by five feet wide, which was a replica of the monolith on a sliding track. The steel plate was a perfect marker for the CSC vault, not bold or gaudy but a work of art.

⟋⟍

About a month after the vault was completed, water started seeping through the walls. We had excessive amounts of waterproof insulation, but it made little difference. Six months after construction, the vault was accumulating a foot of water per day. We spent several hours each day pumping out and mopping up. The room became a haven for black widow spiders, slugs, and snails. Once we found a garter snake swimming among the capsules in the murky mess.

Time passed, and my early hopes faded. The predicted boom in cryonics patients never materialized. I was dumbfounded that we had no new patients who could afford the expense of cryonics. I had taken on too much too soon and made an unwise gamble of trying to save the lives of my friends. I had a state-of-the-art cryogenic capsule capable of holding up to thirty patients. There it was, sitting on a hill in the back of the cemetery just waiting to be used. But timing in so many aspects of life meant the difference between success and failure. For us the timing was bad, and success remained elusive. The huge twenty-four-hundred-gallon vessel was never installed—never used to save the frozen heroes who needed it so desperately.

CHAPTER 7

Lost Hope

Mr. Hope's capsule as presently constructed is too costly and it appears that he hasn't had the money or urge in recent months to improve it, which I suppose is understandable, but I don't relish the idea of rotting in one of his liquid nitrogen containers. I've always thought it appeared to be a portion of a storm drain with each end welded shut.

—Letter from Russ Stanley to Robert Ettinger, dated January 7, 1966

With Frank Farrell's help, I completed the vault. We were now ready to permanently store our patients; however, both the CSC and I were broke. Two years of my life and several thousand dollars had disappeared caring for these people, and now I was out of options. I needed to borrow five hundred dollars from the bank, but I dreaded asking my wife to cosign a loan. My family had suffered through numerous lean years while I dumped my scarce funds into maintaining our frozen friends.

I pulled my car into the driveway at our home, carefully considering my words for this unfair request. I glanced in my rearview mirror and then turned away, unable to look at myself.

When I walked into the house, she knew something was wrong. I was never at home in the middle of the afternoon. I steeled my nerves and plunged into the story.

When I finished, Elaine sat there for five minutes studying her hands. Then she replied in a quiet voice, "This cryonics is ruining our life, ruining our marriage, and consigning me to only half a life. It's put us in poverty, put our kids in jeopardy, and you're asking me for more? My little bit of credit?" She didn't sound accusatory; she was just stating reality.

"Please, I'm desperate. I'm on my knees begging." I took her hands in mine, hoping to convince her. I would sacrifice every last shred of pride to persuade her, but I also knew she loved me, despite everything, and that she wouldn't say no.

She sighed and agreed. We went to the bank together, and she signed. When that money was gone, we were no better off than before.

The 1970 National Cryonics Conference at the Airport Marina Hotel in Los Angeles was fast approaching, and I had planned to give walking tours of the vault. I never told the other cryonics members, but the convention was my last hope. Unfortunately, the Nisco capsule was not holding a vacuum and was wasting liquid nitrogen like a leaky faucet. I didn't have the money to replenish it two to three times per week. We managed to get the vault completed and to install the capsule just a few days before the conference. I tried hiding my desperation both to the people attending the conference and to the other CSC members. Such obvious and blatant need would have invited too many questions.

I showed the vault to Professor Ettinger and several prominent cry-onicists, but no one at the conference offered financial help. Despair was closing in fast! I knew the last few grains of sand were emptying from the hourglass. I could stall with temporary solutions no longer—the permanent lodgings I had hoped for had never developed, and now the permanent solution was likely going to be death. Before I could decide the fate of this failing capsule, I had to take a pilgrimage and reconcile the fate of my dear friends, for I could carry them no more.

My magical Shangri-La was deep in the desert, an oasis free from people and the agonies of life. Planning to stay from sunrise to sunset, I brought a big blanket, several jugs of water, fruit, writing material, and my huge black Belgian shepherd, Bull.

I traveled east out of the San Fernando Valley, passing Magic Mountain and heading toward Palmdale. I turned off the Antelope Valley Freeway for my hidden spot, crossed streams, and traversed miles of barren desert, cruising into oblivion in my beloved red Porsche Speedster. I worried about getting stuck here; however, I knew deep down that nothing bad could happen in this enticing place. I looked over at Bull sitting beside me, nose out the window, black ears flapping in the wind; he was loving every minute of this trek.

I realized I was fighting to preserve experiences like these—this feeling of unbridled, unguarded *life*. I wasn't interested in cryonics for mere survival; it was to provide humanity with as many of these moments as possible. No boundaries should hold people back from the joy of life.

Extended life through cryonics is part of the natural evolution of medicine and could provide a second chance to people, especially the young, whom fate had given an incurable disease. If I were suspended and reanimated centuries from now, I might not have my family by my side anymore, but I would still manage to experience the same joy I found on this day and in this place of solitude. If I were shipwrecked on a deserted island, inexorably separated from my family for the remainder of my life, I would still embrace all the wonders of life.

Dodging the roadrunners, rabbits, and tumbleweeds crossing in front of our vehicle, I traveled about four miles northeast toward the San Gabriel Mountains. The mountains fed a wide creek, flowing strong and fast like a river snake across the desert floor and extending into infinity at the horizon. The beiges and browns of the barren desert transitioned near the creek bank into a verdant paradise lush with small trees, brush, and flowers—as diverse, untouched, and sanctified as Ecuador's Galapagos Islands. After reaching the water, I traveled a half mile upstream to a conglomeration of boulders. Surrounded by the floral aura of an altar, I claimed this place as my very own world. Bull had leapt from the vehicle and dashed into the water; he was gone exploring for hours. We both shared the same excitement generated by the mystery of this glorious place.

I spread out my blanket and waded into the cold, crystal-clear stream for hours; hummingbirds and badgers kept rambling to the creek bank to check on me. After a few hours of feeling the warm sunlight on my face, I allowed my mind to confront the ghastly dilemma of no money and a worn-out, malfunctioning cryo-capsule.

I had always been ruled by emotion—not logic. I was a passionate crusader, not a businessman. In retrospect, if I had said no to a few people and spent my money on a better infrastructure, then all the CSC funds wouldn't have evaporated with the liquid nitrogen and dry ice. I could have built a solid foundation so that I could realistically say yes to later candidates. But those frozen heroes were my friends, and I thought of them as family. Like anyone else, I wanted to fight for my family. And I was an optimist; I had been confident something would succeed for our patients so that my promises could be redeemed. I had been the least-likely candidate for this responsibility. I wasn't a scientist, but fate must've known something. I had relied on that fate to make this work somehow.

The answers came swiftly and clear, carried into my heart, mind, and soul by the gentle summer breeze.

I have to face that this is as far as I can take you, my beloved friends. I have tried with all my might, but I have to let go. I can no longer bear this enormous load alone. Please forgive me.

I was saying good-bye to these friends, and it broke my heart. First I considered Russ Stanley. Russ had accomplished so much to advance the cryonics movement and was an outspoken advocate. However, he left only ten thousand dollars to the society. While that amount was more than anyone else had given, it was insufficient to purchase a good capsule in addition to the maintenance costs. After his death, I had placed him in temporary storage since we had no reliable capsule available; my conscience could see it no other way. We tried our best during those early days. The dry ice replacement for two years cost almost his entire bequest—$9,600—not counting gasoline for the weekly hundred-mile drive.

I remembered a letter he had written to Professor Ettinger in 1966, and it compounded my guilt. Russ wrote: "I don't relish the idea of rotting in one of those liquid nitrogen containers. I've always thought it appeared to be a portion of a storm drain with each end welded shut."

This image he had abhorred was exactly the fate I was trying to reconcile in my mind. I felt like an executioner, condemning him to rot in that capsule because I had failed. Russ had no family and told me he had no one in his life to care.

Next I considered Marie Sweet. I hadn't known Marie very well, but she was a whirlwind of a soul who spent her life fighting for the rights of others. She was a heroine of the women's rights movement. Marie had arranged the first national cryonics conference almost completely by herself. She died without money and, even more disastrously, had been dead two days before she was discovered and cooled down. That fact alone probably sealed her fate.

Again I had to acknowledge the loss, just as for Russ. *This is as far as I can take you, my sweet Ms. Sweet. It was an honor to know you in this lifetime.*

My third patient was Helen Kline, whom I had met at the initial cryonics meeting in 1966. She accomplished so much for a tiny, broke, dying little lady. She never expected to be frozen, although it was her fondest wish. Three weeks before her death, she sent CSC a check for one hundred dollars. It was a parting gift from a precious soul. *Au revoir, sweet lady. You made one hell of a try. You are my hero and an example of what can be accomplished when a person has nothing but faith and a burning desire.*

The final and by far most difficult decision was for Louis Nisco. He was already frozen when I took responsibility for him. His daughter had interred him into one of the first capsules, but she had no place to store the capsule or pay for maintenance. The final deathblow came when his capsule kept failing to keep its vacuum and hold the expensive liquid nitrogen.

Fate had already determined my options. I had always had a revulsion of death, and that sentiment probably motivated my strong devotion to cryonics. For years I had persistent dreams in which I woke up in a coffin. I could see my family crying, but I couldn't speak to them or console them. I always had avoided funerals, with the exception of my stepfather's. Since I'd taken up with cryonics, my dreams had ceased.

I hung my head low, remembering that this wasn't about me but about my four patients. I was killing them and felt sure that my nightmares would return. I trudged out of my pristine Garden of Eden and returned to the cemetery vault, yielding to the Grim Intruder. Now penniless, I had no choice but to watch as the remaining liquid nitrogen boiled off, drop by precious drop, sealing the fate of the friends within. Even if someone had donated a few thousand dollars for liquid nitrogen replacement, it would only have prolonged the agony. I swallowed hard as the last bit of vapor dissipated into the night sky, mortified at the notion that it carried away the spirits of my four friends.

I had witnessed something not required of any human in history: Death had taken my friends twice. This time there was no chance of them coming back. I had fallen short, and I had to accept the responsibility for that failure—alone.

Chapter 8

Newfound Hope

In September 1970 I received a call from brothers Dennis and Terry Harrington, who lived in Des Moines, Iowa. Their mother, Mildred, was dying of cancer, and they wanted to know if she could be frozen. Performing a perfusion in the Midwest intrigued me, but I had several requirements to make this work.

For a ten-thousand-dollar donation, Joseph Klockgether, Professor Ettinger, and I would fly to Iowa, perform the perfusion, ship the body to California, and keep Mildred in temporary storage. Once she was in a capsule, the brothers agreed to pay one hundred to three hundred dollars monthly for the liquid nitrogen until the thirty-patient unit was operational.

I felt wary about trying again after our failure but not yet ready for our cryonics journey to end. Although I was battle weary and scarred from losing my friends, the idea of caring for another frozen body was tempting. I agreed and, once again, jumped into the chasm of the unknown.

When I flew out to meet the brothers and stay at their apartment, I saw they were a curious study in opposites. Terry was effete, with long flowing hair, and worked as a nurse. Dennis was muscular and taught at a karate school. Terry was strong-willed and had initiated their mom's freezing, while Dennis was soft-spoken and often placated his brother. They were identical in one aspect: They dearly loved their mother.

They were engrossed with cryonics, poring through the brochures and making plans to form their own group. Surprisingly, the freezing arrangements went smoothly considering that we were in the middle of the Midwest. I had never been to Iowa, but I always assumed that a place like Des Moines would not receive me or cryonics very well. However, I was happily wrong. Within a few days, I found a cooperating doctor and mortuary.

A week after I arrived, death came in the night for Mildred Harrington. As I submerged her body in ice, Terry closely monitored the procedure to make sure every strand of hair was frozen properly in place. I called Professor Ettinger and Joseph with the unhappy news, and they hopped on planes. The perfusion went smoothly, and the brothers quickly transitioned from heartache to showmanship. The local newscast loved the story of Mildred's suspension, and the Harrington brothers loved the attention. Whenever there was a camera in a crowd, Terry found it.

Among the clamor of microphones and interviews, Joseph Klockgether commented, "These Harrington brothers are media hounds. I don't typically see folks acting like this, even in LA. I'm sure they're grieving, but it seems they care more about publicity than the perfusion."

I waved off Joseph's concerns and smiled. Their mother had been sick for a long time, and I knew everyone grieved differently. I'll admit it was amusing to see Terry sporting a comb and mirror in his back pocket and primping his long hair before stepping into the limelight. He picked out his clothes each morning with such care, trying on several outfits and debating the perfect balance between flamboyance and mourning.

Joseph flew back to Los Angeles to transport Mildred to his mortuary, while I remained at Dennis's apartment for another week. The hospital where Terry worked was hosting a symposium titled "Death and the Dying Process" and invited me to speak about cryonics. Standing at the podium, I felt trepidation and sweaty palms and yet an equal measure of amazement at the paths of life. Here I was, with barely a high-school education, lecturing nearly one hundred physicians about cryonics.

When Terry and Dennis completed the donation paperwork and the seminar was over, I said good-bye to the brothers, wished them well, and returned to LA to commence my weekly ritual of replacing Mildred's dry ice in the vault.

Week after week, Frank Farrell and I accomplished the dangerous, Herculean task of replacing the dry ice. The underground vault had little if any ventilation, and every week we needed to replenish at least three hundred pounds of dry ice, which sublimes into carbon dioxide gas. We pumped out the foot of water that had accumulated during the week on the vault floor. Frank flashed the light in the vault and illuminated the remaining inch of icky, unpumped water with hundreds of floating spider carcasses swirling around Mildred's container.

I knew the dangers; any mistake would be deadly. A single breath of the carbon dioxide would have rendered me unconscious, and Frank would be unable to immediately assist or lift me out of the vault before I asphyxiated. Half-joking, I once told Frank that if I did stumble, he should allow me to stay, as I lay among my friends.

Typically, I went down the ladder into the vault at the cemetery while Frank assisted topside. Darkness shrouded the damp walls and farther recesses of the vault, but I knew crawling spiders were there. After taking several quick breaths, I swallowed my fright, inhaled deeply, rushed down the ladder, and removed the lid of the temporary storage container. Then I scurried back up the ladder, gasping for air. That first trip was merely the prelude to the real work.

I lugged forty pounds of dry ice, cut into four two-inch-thick slices wrapped in thick paper, onto my shoulder. Balancing them, I hurried down to the floor, ripped off the paper, and placed the dry ice into the container. I then scurried up the ladder toward daylight and gasped for air. For eight trips up and down, I repeated that procedure, worried that each trip would be my last. I needed thick gloves to avoid cold burns, but they made it difficult to grip the ladder rungs, making a slip more likely. If I fell, I knew I'd instinctually inhale and then die. When I climbed out of the hole after the final trip, I dropped onto my back on the cemetery grass, regaining my breath, relieved we were done for another week. I never told my wife or my kids about this part of my job for fear that they would insist I quit.

After twenty weeks of that adrenaline-filled terror, we added an emergency scuba rig at the bottom. The spooky vault still resembled a medieval dungeon until we rigged up electric lights and a blower to disperse the suffocating gas. Then our job was more relaxed and I needn't fear for my life each week.

After Mildred had been in temporary storage for two years, the brothers asked if they could hold a two-hour memorial service and a viewing of their mom. This intriguing request provided several challenges, and I was excited to carry out their wishes. I consulted with Joseph, and we designed a special casket with a liquid-nitrogen spray device connected to a thermostat and a spray valve to keep Mildred at low temperature during the service. I knew Mildred was in no danger of thawing during the hours of the memorial, but we didn't want to needlessly worry her sons. The total cost of the service and this special casket was five thousand dollars. The family eagerly set a date.

We purchased an inexpensive casket and tore out the padding, then bought polyurethane insulation for the bottom and sides. Once mixed, these two chemicals, a polyol and an isocyanate, would harden within three minutes and needed to be poured immediately. Those liquids were extremely toxic; I didn't want them around my kids or to let my wife know I was risking my life once again, so I went to the home of a very tolerant friend.

Standing in Mark's garage, I picked up one of the chemical bottles, the isocyanate, emblazoned with several warnings and a skull and crossbones. The liquids emitted a horrible-smelling toxic gas that could kill a person with prolonged exposure. I was amazed at all the life-threatening adventures I'd accumulated with cryonics—the cloak-and-dagger maneuvering with off-kilter clients, the weekly descent into the claustrophobic vault filled with suffocating carbon dioxide, and now exposing myself to what I presumed was cyanide gas. I looked down at the casket and ruefully told myself that if this task poisoned me, then at least I could fall into my final resting place.

I genuflected in my mind and began pouring the chemicals; I soon felt dizzy and nauseated, so we opened the garage door and pulled the casket out into the alleyway to allow the fumes to escape. We finished after an hour and pulled the casket back into the garage; we went into the house and cleaned up. Ten minutes later I heard banging on the front door. Mark was still scrubbing the persistent smell off his hands, so I opened his door and was confronted by four policemen, hands on their holsters.

I obeyed their orders and put up my hands. Mark and I exchanged questioning glances as we got frisked; I hated that feeling of unwelcome hands roving all over my body.

After the search was over, an officer asked, "All right, who's in that coffin you got there in your garage?"

I heaved a sigh of relief and replied, "Come on. We'll show you." They followed us into the garage, and I showed them the empty casket. The almond smell of the noxious gas was still clinging to the polyurethane, and the cops were anxious to return to the alley. I explained that we were working on an experiment and apologized. It never dawned on us what the neighbors might think. We had an uneasy laugh and said good-bye to the police.

Finally the day for the memorial arrived. Santa Ana winds blew in hot temperatures, and I was glad we had taken the extra precaution of the liquid-nitrogen casket. The Harrington brothers managed to amuse me again; Terry was dressed all in white and Dennis all in black. Terry worked diligently on his mother's makeup. I allowed him fifteen-minute intervals to work his magic before closing the lid and turning on the liquid-nitrogen spray. Mildred stayed cold—from her black wig and false eyelashes down to the hem of her embroidered white gown. She had an aura of the fairy-tale princess Sleeping Beauty.

Ten guests attended the viewing. The memorial proceeded just as any other funeral service. It didn't seem to bother anyone that she had been dead for two years—their reaction gave me hope that cryonics would find wider acceptance. Her relatives lingered at the open casket, commenting about how wonderful she looked and that it was such a blessing to see her again. I was content to stand at the back of the chapel in Joseph's mortuary, feeling gratified that I was able to make this day happen.

I overheard a buxom aunt decked out in pink chiffon and swishing a lacy fan say, "Oh, Terry, she's purty as a picture. Your momma was always such a stylish woman. You've done her proud."

One gentleman, obviously a farmer from his tanned, leathery skin and roughened hands, came up to me and said, "You're in charge here right? I remember you from Iowa."

I shook his offered hand and nodded.

"This is some amazing technology you got here. Mildred looks like she closed her eyes forever just an hour ago. What a comfort this must be to the boys, since their momma was such an amazing woman. This all is different from what I'm used to, to be sure. But those brothers are different too. The service suits them."

Dennis and Terry approached me after the memorial, and Dennis gave me a bear hug that cracked my back and lasted several seconds beyond comfortable. He said, "I thank you. This memorial was worth every penny."

I pushed against his muscled chest, released myself from his strong arms, and responded, "I'm glad it was a comfort. Perhaps you've started a new tradition."

Terry's eyes grew wide as though he'd just had a revelation. "Why, yes! I've always wanted to be a trendsetter. Perhaps I've found my calling."

CHAPTER 9

Second Chances

"My daughter has cancer and doesn't have long to live. Can you help?"

That was my first conversation with Guy de la Poterie in July 1971. He was calling from Montreal, Canada, and spoke with a thick French accent. "It's a Wilms tumor. She has already lost one kidney and the other one is failing," he went on to explain. "Her doctors have given up and are simply waiting for her to die."

"*Genevieve's only seven years old.*"

Guy said his family had lost all hope until he saw a news story on TV about cryonics and realized that might be his daughter's only chance. In the news story, a truck signed with Cryonics Society of Michigan had led Guy to Professor Robert Ettinger and then to the Cryonics Society of California.

He wanted Genevieve frozen and suspended when she passed on. I hesitated. "I've never dealt with a hospital outside the United States and have no idea how they'd react. I'd also need the cooperation of a local mortuary."

After hanging up the phone, I stared at the receiver for a long time. This little girl had her entire life ahead—could still have an entire life. If cryonics worked like it should, then someday Genevieve could go to college, perhaps get married and have children of her own. She would die—a clinical death, certainly—but she might still wake up and grow up. This little girl could have a future; I felt intoxicated, overwhelmed. This idea of hope, of possibility, of unscripted futures brought me back to that moment at the beach when I first read Professor Ettinger's book.

I offered to fly to Montreal with Joseph Klockgether and see what arrangements could be made. I told Guy that if he paid the travel expenses, CSC wouldn't charge for our time to come to Montreal. He reserved a hotel room for us and sent two plane tickets. We flew to Canada the next day.

When we arrived in Montreal, Guy stood at the airport gate. He was strikingly trim and good-looking. What struck me most was his gentle and kind eyes, although tired and bloodshot, eloquent reminders of the battle this father had waged. I liked him immediately. Montreal was cool, even in July; the air held a crispness and vitality that was lacking in the lazy Southern California summers. He took us to a comfortable French bistro, filled with the intoxicating aromas of baking baguettes and duck confit, where we settled in for three hours. Since I was to participate in something so personal, I was glad for the opportunity to know him better. Guy knew little about cryonics, and unlike most other people I'd helped, he hadn't been part of the CSC. Despite his inner turmoil, he was able to discuss the logistics objectively.

"We want to help, but you need to fully understand the obstacles. The normal price for performing a perfusion and freezing is ten thousand dollars. That doesn't include the capsule, the monthly maintenance, and liquid-nitrogen replacement fees. We also need investment funds for perpetual care when you and I are no longer here."

He looked as though I had just slapped him. Obviously he hadn't considered the cost. Guy bit his lip and sat there for a long moment holding his coffee cup, elbows planted on the table. "I don't have that kind of money," he finally said, a slight trill in his voice. "I will absolutely find it though. I'll call my parents and my wife's relatives. We'll be good for at least the initial ten thousand dollars."

Wanting to lessen the expenses, I told him Genevieve could double up in another capsule, which would eliminate the monthly fees for liquid nitrogen. This suggestion made him a little squeamish, but he understood. In the meantime, he would need to pay for the dry ice to keep her in temporary suspension.

Piling on the issues, I added, "We also need the assistance of Genevieve's hospital and the local mortuary. We have no idea how these two institutions will react."

"Let me tell you about Genevieve," he said. Absentmindedly, Guy pushed his fork through his mashed potatoes and spoke slowly, as though struggling to find the words to properly describe his beloved daughter, to illustrate that she was extraordinary and yet still a normal little girl.

"She's my youngest. I have two other daughters, whom Genevieve idolizes. She follows them everywhere they go, which is okay with them . . . most of the time. She can't hold still for one minute. She's like a downed high-voltage line, whipping around in fifteen different directions at once. And she likes to tell funny little stories. It's a rare day when she doesn't make us all smile at least once. But so much changed, so much ended for all of us when she got sick."

After we finally said good-bye, I found the hotel and fell onto the bed, recounting my impressions of Guy de la Poterie. No money and no funds, but filled with love. I felt like I was jumping again into the abyss, but I knew this was my duty. No one else would—or could—help them. I heard a light patter of rain against the window, which brought my focus back to the present. I called the hospital and arranged to talk to the director, Mrs. Lemay, the following morning. My last thought before I dozed off was the hope that a woman might be more compassionate than a man.

The next morning, sunlight streamed in through the translucent hotel curtains. Remembering my important mission, I jumped out of bed, flipped the DO NOT DISTURB sign on the door, and rehearsed during a long shower. My presentation was professional and compelling—as long as I had the right audience. However, I was anxious, since I liked Guy and felt connected to his family. I steeled myself and walked to her office.

I explained the cryonics procedure to the director, told her of our past successes, and reiterated that Genevieve's parents strongly desired the suspension. She asked few questions during my ten-minute talk. When finished I awaited her response, twisting my briefcase strap around my hands and trying to gauge her reaction.

Finally she spoke. "The hospital has no policy regarding the preparation of patients for cryonic suspension, and we are strictly regulated by the government. The hospital cannot be involved in cryonics with regards to the girl's case in any way." Her voice sounded clipped and scripted, with a tinge of underlying compassion. Her response left no room to maneuver. "We are discharging her tomorrow, since the doctors can do nothing more. We expect she will live about six more weeks, and her family should simply enjoy every minute the child has left."

Letting out a long sigh, I thanked her for her time and left.

Joseph Klockgether later told me that he had received similar responses from the two mortuaries he contacted. It appeared there was nothing else we could do in Canada.

That evening, we stood in the foyer of the de la Poterie home. Guy and his wife, Pierrette, knew I had bad news the instant they saw my face. They remained silent, disappointed but unsurprised. Pierrette turned away, and Guy dug his hands deep into his pockets, as though resisting the temptation to punch a wall. Feeling profoundly helpless, I just stood there, glancing at the baby pictures filling the room and contemplating other possibilities—other hospitals in Quebec or Ottawa. Several minutes passed before Guy sank into his sofa and looked toward me.

Guy spoke a few sentences in French until he remembered his audience and began again. "Bob, Joe, I'd never heard of a Wilms tumor until the doctor told me that it would kill my daughter. The doctor invited us into his office and told us Genevieve had about a month to live." Guy reached for Pierrette's hand and squeezed it tight. "Simple as that. 'Your daughter has a month.' As if it was as inconsequential as the weather. I suppose to him she was."

Joseph and I said our good-byes and flew home, feeling we couldn't help Genevieve. The problems seemed insurmountable, but five days later Guy surprised me. He was in California, and Genevieve had been accepted into the Children's Hospital in Hollywood. She would fly into Los Angeles with her mother the next day. I was elated at this new opportunity for Genevieve. The situation reminded me of an old saying I had long treasured: "Whether you think you can or you cannot, you are absolutely right."

The next evening at the hospital, I met this little girl I had heard so much about. She was charming, with cropped chocolate-colored hair and big, doe-brown eyes that betrayed her fear and sadness. Though she looked gaunt and tired from the long flight, her apple cheeks looked pink, and she sat up in her hospital bed flanked by her dolls and stuffed animals. Apparently her condition had taken a positive turn.

I requested a meeting with the hospital director the following morning, and to my surprise my call was transferred to him immediately. I didn't have my presentation prepared in that instant but quickly gained my bearings and jumped into the speech I had given in Canada. I wished I could meet with the director in person though; he'd be able to read my character, see my passion and integrity, and feel more comfortable with this girl's unorthodox path. I had to convince him—Genevieve and her parents needed me to succeed.

I explained that I was president of the Cryonics Society of California and that we intended to accept Genevieve as a medical donor, which was her father's wish. Therefore, we needed to pack her body in ice and administer a shot of heparin immediately upon clinical death.

After a brief pause the director asked, "You're the organization that freezes people, right?"

My stomach jumped. I had no choice but to be honest. "Well, I suppose you could put it that way."

He told me to hold for a moment . . . about twenty minutes clicked by in total silence.

"I'm sorry that took so long." The director stopped to clear his throat. "I just spoke with the hospital supervisor. She'll provide you with anything you need and cooperate in every way possible."

My heart quickened and I bounced in the chair, nearly speechless with this change in fortune.

"Furthermore, if you have any problems or need anything else, just call me back."

He gave me his personal pager number, and I thanked him countless times. What a difference from my experience in Montreal! I couldn't wait to tell Genevieve's family. God knew they needed some good news.

Still elated, I had to switch my mind back to the logistics, such as finding a place near the hospital where Genevieve's parents could stay. Their plan was for each of them to stay one week, rotating so that one of them would be home to care for their other two children. The cost for a small, one-bedroom apartment near the hospital was astronomical. On the third day of searching, we found one that they could reasonably afford.

The first week Guy stayed and his wife went home. I met with him almost every day. He was elated when I told him about the hospital's enthusiastic offer of cooperation.

He couldn't get the ten thousand dollars from his family, so I found myself accepting another cryonic suspension without being paid for it. But saying no to that beautiful child was simply not an option.

Each morning when I arrived at the hospital, I'd stand in the doorway of Genevieve's room, watching her play nurse to her dolls. After all her time in hospital beds, she knew the job description quite well. She pretended taking their temperature, withdrawing blood from the squishy doll arms with a tiny straw, and placing cold compresses on their little foreheads. The big nurses would constantly come in with big needles—needles for injecting something into the little girl or taking fluids out. Brave Genevieve scrunched up her face and steeled herself, but she never cried or jerked her arm, not even making a soft whimper. The nurses acted sweet but spoke in this high-pitched affected tone that adults often take with children.

Pierrette returned to relieve Guy the following week for the next rotation. I watched Pierrette tend to her daughter, endlessly smoothing her hair, arranging her blankets, and soothing her with stories, trying to fit a lifetime of mothering into the next few short days. I caught the names of Genevieve's brother and sister, but since they were speaking in French, I couldn't understand much else. As a mother, Pierrette was in agony, but with Genevieve she was always cheerful and smiling.

I was struck again by how strongly this family was committed to the hope that cryonics provided. These parents, by alternating weeks, were forfeiting precious days and memories so that Genevieve could be here in

California—with me. One of them probably wouldn't be here at the end. Watching their sacrifice of a parent's most precious commodity—time— strengthened my resolve that their efforts would not be in vain.

After her brief reunion with Genevieve, Pierrette turned to me and said, "Mr. Robert, my daughter has a question."

"Of course," I replied. "I'm here and at her service."

She looked pleased as her mom translated for me, though she didn't smile. Pierrette, combing her fingers through her daughter's hair, looked at me. "Genevieve wants to know if you know where Disneyland is."

"Well, of course," I responded, nodding. "That's where my old friends Mickey Mouse and Donald Duck live."

After the translation, exhilaration filled her face until she glowed. The excited girl asked, "You really know them?"

"Oh, yeah. We go back a long way." I turned to Pierrette and asked, "Is there any chance we can go?"

A smile dawned, erasing all traces of Pierrette's exhaustion. "The doctor agreed. He said it would be far preferable than sitting here all day." Pierrette glanced at all the machines, one constantly drawing a red line on a strip chart. "I think she's strong enough if we use a wheelchair and carry her whenever possible."

I asked Genevieve if we could go to Disneyland tomorrow to meet Mickey and Donald. I watched, delighted, as the little girl's eyes grew wider and wider. Sadly though, she did not smile, just clapped her hands.

When I arrived home that night, I wrapped my nine-year-old daughter, Susan, in a big hug. "Can you do a big favor for daddy?" I asked.

"Of course," she answered, placing her hand on my cheek.

"I want you to skip school tomorrow."

She leaned back, giving me a skeptical look. "Skip school?" she asked, surprised that would be an option, let alone a favor. "You'd let me skip school?"

I smiled. "This is something super special for a very special little girl. She doesn't have too many chances for fun times. So can you help me make sure she has lots of fun tomorrow?"

Nodding, Susan realized this was important grown-up business.

"We're going to Disneyland tomorrow."

Thrilled, she jumped up and spun around and round. "Wow, best favor ever!"

The drive to Disneyland was enchanting. Genevieve and her mom never stopped talking. She pressed her face against the car window and squealed "*Maman, Maman!*" when she first glimpsed the Sleeping Beauty Castle from the freeway. It was tough for me to drive; I kept wanting to look in the rearview mirror and watch her excitement grow as she spoke faster and faster. When we arrived we picked up a wheelchair and a special pass for Genevieve's condition.

We went straight to It's a Small World, my personal favorite, and since it's a boat ride, I knew it wouldn't be too taxing on Genevieve. She loved it so much she insisted we go around three times, pointing out the Eiffel Tower each time. I realized something deeply poignant while sharing the Small World ride with her. Whether American, Canadian, French, or Japanese, children all over the world have the same innocence and bestow dreams and possibility on a weary world. Just as cryonics brings hope to an individual, children—the next generation—provide hope for all humanity.

For the next couple of hours, we strolled through Fantasyland, a medieval fair with gentle rides. Genevieve seemed free of her life-and-death drama. When we came to the teacups, she asked her mom to ride with her. Before that, Susan had accompanied her on the rides. Her mom flashed me a funny look as she boarded. I think the ride made her a little nervous. Wrapped in the blanket, Genevieve appeared as small as Alice after she drank from the bottle in Wonderland. As the teacups spun around, I watched the blurry girl gripping the teacup rim; a few stray hairs blew wildly. When the ride ended, I scooped her up and placed her back in the wheelchair. She was breathless but had excited eyes and rosy cheeks.

"Mr. Robert," Pierrette said. "Genevieve wants me to ask you a question."

"Please, go right ahead and ask."

"Genevieve wants to know if you would learn French so that she can talk with you."

I knelt down and looked into those beautiful brown eyes and said, "Genevieve, I will learn French just for you."

As her mother translated, Genevieve enchanted me with a big precious smile, the only smile I ever saw on her face during the time I knew her. When her mom told me that was also the first smile she had seen since Genevieve had become ill, I had an idea. Genevieve needed to meet two individuals who had no shortage of smiles—Mickey and Donald.

I slipped away while the children rode the charming horses on the King Arthur Carrousel. I went on a hunt for someone who could send Mickey and Donald our way. I was eventually guided toward the park director, a young lady with black hair, a lovely smile, and compassionate eyes, reminding me of Snow White.

I explained Genevieve's situation, and she grabbed my hand. "Anything Genevieve wants to see is hers for the asking."

"Could Mickey and Donald sort of bump into us?"

Patting me on the back, she called on her walkie-talkie; in five minutes everything was prepared.

She flashed a smile and leaned in close, as if delivering a top-secret mission. "Stroll over to the Casey Jones train ride close to the water fountain at noon. Mickey and Donald will run up to you like you're long-lost brothers."

A fire lit inside me. Genevieve was going to be thrilled!

I didn't say anything to Pierrette or my Susan. I just meandered our group over to the train station at eleven forty-five.

Genevieve had asked her mom twice that morning about Mickey and Donald. It was one minute before noon, and my heart was racing. Genevieve looked at me, about to ask something, when the magic happened. Genevieve's face lit up; she bounced in her wheelchair, waving and yelling in French.

Of course I knew exactly what was happening but pretended I didn't see anything. She gestured wildly at our approaching guests. "Monsieur Robert, look! Look!"

When I turned around, Donald tackled me, capturing me in a big hug as I accidentally stepped on his big duck feet. Mickey joined him about two seconds later. It was perfect; my smile was as wide and permanent as Mickey's. Genevieve was so excited she was close to tears. I settled my two long-lost buddies down and introduced them to the girls. My daughter had figured out the charade, but she played along flawlessly.

We settled down on a grassy knoll with a bench far from the crowds. Susan and I stepped away, allowing Genevieve and her mom to enjoy those two characters, so adept at providing a magical spark to a child's life. As Genevieve's mom interpreted what the Disney characters were saying, the girl's imagination took her far away from the hospitals, doctors, and needles. I was happy that Pierrette had allowed me to bring along a movie camera to capture it all on film. I knew that all too soon, the footage of this extraordinary day would be precious to Genevieve's family. After visiting for about thirty minutes, Donald and Mickey indicated it was time to go. Genevieve hugged them for a long moment, scrunching up her face, trying not to cry. The characters shook my hand as they went off, continuing the pretense. However, I was so grateful for Genevieve's happiness and for their gentle compassion that they really were now my best buddies. Genevieve chirped happily with her mom, reliving the experience and rides.

I adopted her in my heart in that moment. I could not let her or her family down. I swore to myself that she would somehow be placed in cryonic suspension, even if I had to do it all myself. I closed my eyes, pained by all the heartache that fate had brought to this beloved, gentle girl. I could deny her nothing.

As I drove back to the hospital that afternoon, with the fading sun streaming through my side window, I knew that day would live in my memory forever, pristine and golden. I looked back and saw Genevieve in her mother's arms, soft mews coming from her as she slept.

When I visited her in the hospital several days later, she still chatted excitedly about her time at Disneyland, but she looked quite pale and lethargic. I felt the stale hospital air and ghostly white walls and cabinets close around her; the setting was so different from the vibrant colors and squealing voices surrounding her just a few days earlier.

Guy was back, and Pierrette had returned to Canada. Whispering with a hitch in his voice, he told me he had just met with the doctors and decided not to put her on dialysis when her remaining kidney failed. The cancer had returned from its brief remission, and Guy reasoned that within a week she would experience severe pain; it would soon become unbearable and ultimately dialysis would be pointless. The alternative was uremic poisoning; Genevieve would simply go to sleep.

The next three weeks were depressing beyond description. This sweet angel was slipping away, and we could do nothing except comfort her and watch her fade. It was so unfair that I'd outlive that little girl. I just couldn't stop thinking about it. *Is she scared? She doesn't act scared, but how can she not be? Does she truly realize everything this cancer is taking from her—her first dance with a boy, getting to grow up, seeing the actual Eiffel Tower?*

I hoped that cryonics would give her those opportunities—all those experiences would still be hers, just delayed for a little while. If she must go to sleep and be placed in those cold liquids, then please let her wake up later. Heaven can wait—it'll still be there for her after she's had a long, full life.

At night I would go home exhausted and emotionally spent. All I could do was gather my own children into my arms, kiss their hair, and give long hugs until they pulled away.

The doctors told us Genevieve had been in total kidney failure for nine or ten days. The longest they had seen a person survive in that condition was eight days. She had a remarkably strong will to live. By this time Guy had become reclusive, speaking only to Genevieve.

On the tenth day, she was weak and pale, but her eyes were alert as she talked with her dad. On the eleventh day she began to dim rapidly. The end came on the twelfth day. She was holding her daddy's hand when she asked him to hold her. Guy climbed onto the bed and cradled her in his arms. I had just arrived, and as I walked into the room, I stopped and quietly backed out. I couldn't interrupt this moment. I watched through the small window in the door as this gentle father softly rocked his little girl back and forth and stroked her sweet face.

After about twenty minutes, he lay her back down, and I quietly reentered the room. Guy turned to me and said, "Please get a doctor; I believe she has just passed away." He ran his large hand over her small face, closing her eyes.

Within two minutes Genevieve de la Poterie was pronounced legally dead. As we had asked, the nurses immediately covered her tiny body with ice and started the cardiac heart massage machine. Guy trudged down the hallway to a bank of pay phones. Pierrette needed to know.

Genevieve was transported to Joseph Klockgether's mortuary, where we performed an excellent perfusion. We then placed her on dry ice in temporary storage until I could transfer her to a capsule. In her favorite dress and with her lips swollen from the perfusion, she didn't look dead to me, only asleep . . . for now. The perfusion was filmed by a professional cameraman and later used in a documentary.

With my work completed and nothing left to do except keep her forever cold, the full weight of Genevieve's death now came upon me. She had traveled to Hamlet's undiscovered country, the place from which no one had returned—yet. I bowed my head and pressed my face against my fist, covering my eyes and nose. Trying not to make a sound, I gritted my teeth and felt the tightness in my throat. I had to be strong and steel myself against death; I had seen it many times before, but this one was the hardest and ripped at my heart. Today, as I write this, Wilms disease is no longer fatal. Within my own lifetime, medicine has found a cure for what killed that little girl.

My mind had to shift from the horrendous drama of watching Genevieve die to the physical labor of caring for her. Her parents' work was done; they had loved her and cared for her completely. Now it was my turn. Genevieve remained in the temporary storage of a container filled with dry ice alongside Mildred for about a year.

Our fledgling cryonics facility was limping along but slowly gaining strength, and I was determined to make it succeed. Feeling confident about the CSC trajectory, I went back to educating the general public about cryonics. Genevieve and our other frozen heroes were counting on me.

Chapter 10

The East Coast Cryotorium

CRYONIC SOCIETIES WERE SPROUTING UP IN SEVERAL CITIES, mostly on the East and West Coasts. After we had frozen the first man, several other groups, including the Cryonics Society of New York, had followed our lead and frozen some patients as well. I would learn over time that these cryonics societies experienced many of the same problems we did. In March 1971 I received a call from Pauline Mandell, who lived in the Bronx in New York. Her son, Steven, had died of cancer in his early twenties and had been in cryonic suspension at CSNY since 1968. She pleaded with me to come to New York to discuss moving her son to California for long-term storage. Like most other patients held by CSNY, her son's capsule was on the verge of being evicted from Mount Washington Cemetery. She was battling Curtis Henderson, president of CSNY, and their dealings had turned ugly.

Since I was traveling to Boston to visit my ailing mother, I decided to make the side trip to see Pauline, arriving on a beautiful spring day. Since New York City seems to prefer to play at the extremes of temperature, this was one of the few visits when I actually enjoyed the weather. As I emerged from the plane, I saw Pauline waiting on the tarmac, wearing a tan leather jacket and brown jeans like she promised.

She was in her late thirties with a pretty and welcoming face, but her troubles showed in her tired eyes. She pulled out of our hug and began wringing her hands, saying, "Thank you so much for coming. Getting frozen was my son's dying wish. I've tried, but I'm at my wits' end with Mr. Henderson. He made all kinds of assurances and now we're in a big mess.

The management of the cemetery where the capsules are stored wants them out. They've threatened to block delivery of liquid nitrogen if they aren't removed immediately. Mr. Henderson has nowhere to put them. Please, for the sake of my only son, help me fix this."

A lump in my throat made it difficult to speak, so I just patted her shoulder. Her son had been in college with his entire life ahead of him. He deserved a chance.

I noticed a muscular, balding man beside her in his mid-forties, with a tough chiseled face and squinty eyes. She introduced him as Nick DeBlasio and explained that his wife, Ann, was in cryonic suspension and that he was also sparring with Curtis Henderson at CSNY. Nick told me he was a New York City policeman and didn't take any shit from anyone—I believed him.

Nick claimed Curtis had treated him rudely during a discussion about his wife's safety. Apparently things turned ugly when Nick said he found a cigarette butt floating in the liquid nitrogen of his wife's capsule that was the same brand Curtis smoked. I found this hard to believe, but I wasn't going to argue with a cop.

"I ought to sue them or send some of my buddies from the force. They can't go around disrespecting folks, especially my lovely, amazing wife."

I had always known Curtis and the entire CSNY crew to be honest people, and I could not understand all this animosity. I was unprepared to deal with two frozen patients, but I soon learned that Nick didn't want to transfer his wife to California. He wanted his own facility—one in which he alone could take care of his wife and no one else could have access.

"Nick, it took me two years to find a cemetery in California that allowed frozen bodies to be stored on their grounds," I said. "I have no idea how difficult it will be to duplicate a vault for cryonic storage in New York. You know that the cemetery used by CSNY is trying to kick them out."

Nick begged me to try. "I cannot lose my wife; she was my soul mate, the song of my heart, the love of my life."

I realized then that he needed cryonics because he had always used his strength or his strength of will to control situations. Cryonics was a way for him to continue that control even in the face of death. No one and nothing was going to beat him.

"I need to visit my mother, so while I'm gone, choose three possible cemeteries. I'll come back in one week and stay five days." I patted him on the shoulder. "I'll do what I can."

Nick agreed. *Who knows? We might just get lucky.* I was experienced working with cemeteries; at least I could get him pointed in the right direction.

The next week I returned to New York, and Nick handed me a list of three local cemeteries. I sat down at his desk and called his first choice, Mount Holiness Memorial Park in Butler, New Jersey, close to his New York police beat. I explained that I was interested in purchasing land at their cemetery. In less than a minute, John Lewis, the park manager was on the phone. After conjuring up several presentations, I decided to just pitch the truth.

"I represent CSC, a medical research foundation in California conducting experiments in low-temperature biology, and we wish to construct an underground vault to store frozen human remains." I was glad my voice projected some confidence that I certainly did not feel.

"Do you have any other such facilities?" he asked.

I told him about our vault in Chatsworth and then waited through a long pause, not knowing what to expect. Nick swatted me, wanting to know details, and I waved him off. He harrumphed and paced the floor. I was getting irritated with his distracting me; if preparations were as complicated here as in California, he'd be exasperating to handle.

Finally the manager answered, "I hope we can help you. Why don't you come, and we'll see if we can find you a spot."

I was stunned at the open invitation by the first cemetery we called— it was unreal! I asked Nick when he'd like to go.

He jumped off the ground, "Now! Now! Now!" He grabbed his car keys and barreled for the door.

On our drive to Butler, we passed rolling green hills and reveled in the smell of recent rain—so different from the LA sprawl—and it made me nostalgic for my New England childhood. The verdant cemetery was as lush as the surrounding countryside, and the grounds were as manicured as I had ever seen.

I introduced Nick to John Lewis as my East Coast cryonics director who would oversee the facility's operation. John questioned us about the frequency of the liquid nitrogen servicing and how long it took to offload the delivery truck. I responded about once a month and less than half an hour to refill the capsule. Those answers seemed acceptable to him.

He then took us on a tour of the grounds. Nick favored a location close to the entrance, since it would be accessible for the liquid nitrogen truck. We asked to buy that parcel, and I wrote a check from my personal account for five thousand dollars, hoping it wouldn't clear until I called Elaine and she got funds into the bank. We shook hands and said goodbye. I was in shock. This deal had been so easy compared with the grueling rejection from numerous cemeteries I had encountered in California. This good omen was a promising start for Nick's vault.

Nick and I wanted to leave everything at the cemetery under CSC ownership. If all went smoothly for a few months, I would turn the deed and facility over to him and he'd reimburse my expenses.

I told Nick that after we had built our California vault, I found a company with facilities all over the country that installed prefabricated units for a reasonable price. The next morning I called the manufacturer, and we decided on a ten-by-fifteen-foot structure. I called John at the cemetery and arranged to have the ground dug out to accommodate our vault. Nick slapped my back, giddy at our good luck.

Two days later we were at the cemetery, soaking in the crisp spring air. Life—that is, birds and squirrels—flitted all around us. Unlike many other people, I never felt forlorn at cemeteries. Instead I had the dual emotions of hope in the future and disappointment that so many people had gone needlessly into the ground.

At eleven forty-five, an eighteen-wheel truck arrived hauling an enormous double concrete block and a crane. We waved the driver to the right spot, and he hopped out of his cab. Nick and I sat on a stone bench, enthralled by the ensuing well-choreographed performance.

Three burly men built the huge vault in three stages, starting with a bottom slab. Once the crane had that in place, the upper perimeter was coated with a six-inch-thick rubbery, tar-like substance. This goo served as a gasket for the second concrete piece, which formed the sides. When that in turn was lowered, a second tarry gasket was applied to its upper edge in preparation for the top section. Throughout the entire procedure, Nick and I exchanged amazed glances. Within thirty minutes, the vault was in the ground. Since the Chatsworth vault had required two weeks for the main construction, I had hoped this vault would be finished by the weekend—not by lunchtime!

Within forty-five minutes the truck was returning to its home base. Already the groundskeepers were covering the installation with dirt and sod. It was like some fantastic conjuring trick performed on television.

As we left our new East Coast cryonic storage facility, I suggested we meet with Pauline Mandell for an early dinner. Nick took us to a restaurant with the best Chinese cuisine I'd ever had. During the meal I had a brilliant idea that would surely thrill both Pauline and Nick.

"Nick, you could place Pauline's son in the vault with your wife. We could remove Steven from his leaky, rickety capsule and double them up in the new Minnesota Valley Engineering (MVE) unit. There's plenty of space, and it would lower your expenses significantly."

Neither made a sound. They stared at me like I had asked to dig up Stalin and place him in Ann DeBlasio's capsule.

Although it was clear that Nick didn't want any man near his wife, I still tried to convince him. "Nick, you may not think much of it now, but as time goes by, expenses mount; another person can make all the difference."

Pauline sat there frozen with her mouth open, so Nick spoke. "No way that'll ever work. After everything I've been through with those . . . jokers at CSNY, I don't want any complications. That vault is for my wife only. I wouldn't let anyone share it in a million years."

Pauline shook out of her stupor and stood up, her palms supported on the table, "No! I've already had all the problems I can handle. I love my son with all my heart, but I just can't do this anymore."

Pauline was almost shouting, and I could feel the stares from the patrons and the ladies with the dim sum carts. I abandoned my plan. "Of course Pauline; it was just an idea. Silly, really; everything's fine."

She took a deep breath and sat down, but her fluttering hands sent the hot green tea airborne. It spilled across the table, and we ended our dinner quickly after that, my fortune cookie unopened.

I was scheduled to leave the next morning for my return to California, so I needed to think fast. After everything I'd seen of Pauline's behavior, should I commit to flying Steven Mandell's fifteen-hundred-pound capsule to California and add it to my long list of nonpaying suspensions?

I tried talking with Pauline, but she just couldn't focus, preferring instead to shuffle through the papers on her desk or wring her hands while she stared at Steven's photos. I couldn't judge her harshly though. She was generally a nice and professional woman, but her son's death was just far too traumatic.

That evening I stayed at Pauline's home and slept on the problem. By sunrise I was certain she was no longer able to deal rationally with her son's suspension.

However, I just couldn't say no.

If Steven's capsule was operating okay, I could place Mildred and Genevieve in it. Before I could do that, though, I needed her full authorization. I told Pauline that if she donated Steven's body and the capsule to the CSC and paid for transport to California, I would continue his suspension. I carefully explained that my eventual goal was to place all patients, including Steven, in the thirty-person capsule we had purchased. Pauline said she would have to end her son's suspension otherwise, so I had her blessing. I also asked that she make a monthly donation to CSC of one hundred dollars for liquid nitrogen replacement.

Pauline and I needed to find a carpenter to make the special heavy-duty shipping crate for Steven's flight. I never mentioned to the airline that Steven was inside. When the capsule arrived at the Los Angeles airport, I picked it up with a rented truck and brought it directly to the heavy-equipment yard at the Chatsworth cemetery. I did not place it in the vault because I needed easy access to assess its performance.

A year later I returned to New Jersey and was astounded by the transformation of Nick's vault. It had wall paneling, drapes, and fragrant white roses and was painted ivory and robin's egg blue. He'd even brought in a chair so that he could visit comfortably with his wife, and he had asked a monsignor to bless the vault. During a delightful three-course Italian meal at Nick's home that night, he paid me and I transferred ownership of the vault to him.

I lost contact with Pauline. Once her son was in California, she never inquired about him other than a single letter wishing us well. I think for her own survival she needed to walk away from Steven's suspension and the hell she had endured trying to honor his wishes.

Nick took meticulous care of his wife's capsule over the next several years. I always marveled at Nick's duality—he was gruff and bullying but also loving and gentle. He eventually did add another person to Ann's capsule; a woman whom the CSC froze and shipped to him to store and share expenses. In our monthly newsletter I proclaimed that our latest patient was shipped to "our East Coast facility"—a proclamation that I later took a lot of grief over.

Finally bad luck caught up with Nick. The monthly removal of the capsule lid for liquid nitrogen replacement caused an ice layer to form around the lid seat. The ice made it harder and harder to dislodge this top portion. Each time Nick needed to add liquid nitrogen, it was a battle. He began prying the lid off and then used a hammer to bang it off. Finally the capsule developed a microscopic vacuum leak. A capsule with a vacuum leak can no longer function. The liquid nitrogen acted like water in a scalding sauté pan and quickly evaporated.

He attempted to repair the leak a few times, but disaster struck. One day Nick went to top off the liquid nitrogen, but it had long since evaporated. The capsule had been warm for weeks, and his wife had decomposed badly. It was heartbreaking; installing a simple input tube on the capsule for adding more liquid nitrogen could have avoided the ice problem and prevented the tragedy.

The sad end of Nick's beloved wife Ann and the other occupant was truly touching and sobering. He did everything possible to keep them in suspension, hoping to rejoin Ann someday, but there can never be a single mistake—not for hundreds of years.

CHAPTER 11

I Needed the Money

An intriguing New Yorker named Mary Goodman phoned me. She was interested in cryonic suspension upon her death and hoped I could spend a day with her.

The lady's words rolled out silky and proper; she sounded like royalty but with an American accent. "I have been following cryonics for several years, and I want to investigate this as an option for myself," she said.

I agreed to travel to New York if she paid for my time and expenses. She offered five thousand dollars. This princely sum blew me away; I was so broke I thought the phone call was a gift from God.

Ten days later I landed in New York and checked into the Manhattan Towers on 42nd Street. I was nervous and excited about meeting this generous lady. From her Park Avenue address, Mary Goodman was obviously wealthy and could be a benefactor.

At noon I arrived at her building; it was elegant beyond all expectations. The doorman noticed me, my chin high in the air as I gawked at the treasures surrounding me. I gave him my name, and his quizzical expression transformed to a smile.

"Madam is expecting you," he replied with a curt bow, then escorted me through a palatial lobby with pink marble walls and a glittering chandelier high overhead to the golden penthouse elevator. As the doors opened onto her floor, a lady wearing a black satin dress and pearls was waiting. She was an attractive woman for her age, her beauty accentuated by her wealth and sophistication. She offered her fragile hand, adorned with an emerald-cut diamond ring as wide as her knuckle. I shook it gently as she gestured me to follow.

Her parlor was as imposing and imperious as a museum. My house could fit inside this room, and the walls soared to twenty feet overhead, allowing the sunlight and the surrounding city to envelop me. It was full of irreplaceable art objects, including marble busts, crystal vases, and several portraits. Woefully ignorant about art, I avoided giving an opinion on the paintings and sculptures, commenting instead on the magnificent skyline that surrounded us. The view from a wide expanse of windows overwhelmed me like the initial throes of puppy love—it was so unexpected and enthralling. The summits of so many skyscrapers backed by the Hudson River reminded me of the tree canopy in a verdant rain forest. Living at such a vantage point was a heavenly privilege reserved for a lucky few.

I ripped my attention away from the view and back to my hostess. After our introductions, we sat down to tea served with what I believe were crumpets. I had never seen them before, but they reminded me of small English muffins. Channeling memories of playing tea with my daughters, I pretended to enjoy those crumpets, but I really did find them nasty little things.

Clearing my throat to fight off my nervousness, I began. "To what do I owe the pleasure of this meeting?" I cringed a little, hoping I sounded refined instead of someone playacting a role.

Mary sat up straight, her posture impeccable. Her finishing school classes had been many years ago, but she still carried the lessons with her. Her demeanor put me at ease though; she was warm, refined, and polite without a hint of pretension. "I believe this may be a preferred choice to burial or cremation," she said. "I find it exciting that the science of the future could cure all diseases and return frozen people to a new life."

She said that in a careful, prepared way, indicating she had memorized her statements and further assuring me her intentions were serious. I was impressed and told her so.

"You see, Mr. Nelson, I have followed the cryonics movement for some time now, from the shadows. I chose to speak to you because you froze the first man."

I stapled on my sincere smile and said, "That is my purpose for being here. What would you like to know?"

She started with a rather curious question: "Have any famous or very wealthy people been frozen?"

I stopped swishing my spoon around my teacup and replied, "To the best of my knowledge, no. Probably the closest we came to a celebrity suspension was the late Walt Disney."

She grew wide-eyed, and I knew I had her attention. "A Disney representative made this inquiry in 1966 before we froze Dr. Bedford. I told her we didn't have the necessary infrastructure at that time and that I regretted I couldn't give better answers to her questions. If things had worked out differently, Walt Disney could have been the first man frozen. Just imagine where the cryonics movement might be today."

Unfortunately I could only recount our modest accomplishments. "Since the Disney inquiry, we have frozen several people and developed a cryonic storage facility in California, along with a private facility in New Jersey." I gave her a meager list of doctors and scientists working with us.

"What evidence can you offer that cryonics may someday fulfill its promise?" she asked.

I smiled; she had some good questions mixed in with the silly ones. "I think the big question is whether life is static or dynamic. For me everything depends on that answer. Does life require a constant supply of spiritual energy to maintain its existence, or can that energy become latent during unlivable conditions? If so, can the same be replicated in humans? Several animals such as the marmot go dormant for months and then turn life on again when conditions improve. I think of life as something akin to a movie reel. Life energy does not vanish forever when the movie projector is turned off—it can still be recovered.

"From looking at nature, I am hopeful and optimistic. Numerous insects, fish, amphibians, and reptiles freeze for months each winter. These creatures demonstrate that life can be shut down by low temperature until a warmer, friendlier environment returns. Suspending biological activity has saved many species from extinction."

I continued with evidence that had captivated me, mentioning one of my favorite authorities, the well-known and imaginative Russian scientist V. A. Negovskii. In his experiments he brought hundreds of animals to the brink of clinical death and then resuscitated them to a normal, healthy life. The capstone of his life's work, *Resuscitation*, provided lucid comments that certainly apply to human beings: "Death is due to the disturbance of vital mechanisms with irreversible changes in living matter, which disintegrates and decomposes. If the mechanism of life remains intact and its basic structure is not affected, then a complete cessation of life is possible which is not equivalent to death. For life can be restored by a change to more favorable conditions."

Mary was spellbound. After another half hour, she suggested a lunch break. Her cook produced a startling array, including pâté and chateaubriand. Over lunch our conversation diverted to lighter topics.

Her question following lunch was whether she could guarantee to have money in the future. I explained that this was a major concern. "The law allows people to bequeath money for a 'life-in-being plus ninety-nine years.' The life-in-being means you choose a trustee, and after that person's death, the ninety-nine-year period of the trust commences. Of course logic dictates choosing a young, healthy person. There are other alternatives, but they are more complicated."

Her following questions were trivial. "What if I don't like the future? What if I am lonely?"

I indulged her and discussed her concerns by sharing an interview I had done on a television show.

"The host asked if I was married. I replied, 'Yes.' Then he asked, 'What if you died within the year and were frozen and revived fifty years later. Your wife is now eighty and you are thirty, what are you going to do?' I answered simply, 'Get a divorce.'"

Mary patted my hand and said, "I feel for your wife."

I smiled back. "No one is saying everything will be perfect—that's not the nature of life. Life is full of challenges. As Professor Ettinger has often said, 'It's more interesting to be alive than dead.'"

Reveling in my impressive surroundings, I tried a different tack—one I hoped would reach her heart. "Mrs. Goodman, you obviously appreciate beautiful and valuable art. After you are gone, I'm sure you wouldn't want to see these priceless paintings tossed into a fire."

She drew back, startled at the suggestion.

"You also are a radiant woman with so much to offer, and yet people think nothing of having themselves cremated. The life of every good person is a work of art. Just like these sculptures and paintings, such beauty as I see here," I cupped her chin in my hand and looked into her eyes, "should be preserved. That is my life's goal."

Mary gazed around the room at her accoutrements, studying them with a fresh perspective. I knew I had reached her, so I forged ahead. "Just as you value art and want to see it appreciated, I value the potential of future technology and abhor the idea of people needlessly going into the ground or the fire." I gestured to a portrait of a young woman, but I couldn't tell if she wore Victorian or Elizabethan dress. "Look at this lady. She is stunning, and a painter immortalized her on canvas. We can see something of who she was; however, the painting is just a two-dimensional facade. This isn't her, and we know nothing of her. Now just imagine if the technology had existed then to cryogenically preserve this lady in the portrait so that she could know the future and future generations could know her. Just imagine the potential and excitement of that! We now have the power to immortalize our very selves, not just in the things we leave behind or in an image made in oils or in stone but ourselves—our memories, our minds. While art indirectly preserves the products and trappings of our minds, cryonics is the next logical step. It allows us to preserve life itself, the essence of our existence."

We had been talking for several hours, and she asked if I would join her for dinner. I was delighted by her invitation, and we agreed that I would return to my hotel, rest a little, dress, and she would collect me at seven.

Finally I asked her what her thinking was about cryonic suspension. She replied that she definitely saw its logic but needed to speak to some cryobiologists before proceeding. She was bothered that these experts were so strongly opposed to cryonics.

I never heard from her again. I was dismayed and suspected that the long reach of the cryobiologists' cynicism had won over in her mind.

In later years, I received a small income from cosmetic preservation and storage that helped me fund the nonpaying suspensions for some time. Laura Coronel wanted to preserve the body of her father, Pedro Ladesma, not for reanimation but for some mysterious reason I was never able to learn.

Laura looked Hispanic, with straight black hair to her shoulders, and she always wore very expensive, hand-embroidered outfits. During our meetings she needed to take charge, continuously talked over me, and often seemed not to be listening to me at all.

While her sincerity and love for her father could never be questioned, I certainly wondered about her clearness of mind. Pedro Ladesma had been autopsied and embalmed and had remained for six months in cold storage at Forest Lawn Cemetery. My best guess was that his freezing was simply a cosmetic preservation for some political reason back in his native country.

My first meeting with Laura was so bizarre that I debated accepting her father into the Chatsworth vault. However, my patients needed me and I needed her money, so I ignored the peculiarities. She refused to meet at my office or any public location. Instead she gave exotic instructions to meet on a little street off Wilshire Boulevard in Los Angeles.

I waited about twenty minutes at the street corner before she pulled up slowly in her car and waved me over to her window. She handed me a piece of paper with instructions to go to a second location and wait. After ten minutes at the second spot, she drove by slowly while I looked around for anything suspicious, growing more paranoid each passing moment. These were techniques I remembered from my stepfather's mobster days. After a few more minutes, she raced up to my Porsche and hopped in, slamming down the lock button.

"Drive! Drive!"

Instinctually, my foot hit the gas. She committed a scant second to smoothing her hair before she devoted her energy to barking directions of right, left, right while scanning the road for trailing cars. When she sidled next to me to look in the rearview mirror, her expensive perfume was overwhelming.

I hoped all this danger was merely her delusions.

Laura's last direction was to turn right from a left-turn lane. I ignored the honking cars and worried about the real possibility of police sirens behind me. After twenty minutes of this craziness, she finally instructed me to stop in a grocery store parking lot. For some time I white-knuckled the gear shift, feeling light-headed from such a sustained adrenaline rush.

I started slowly, "I've got to know about all this cloak-and-dagger maneuvering."

She leaned in and whispered, "I need to be very careful, since my father was a very important man. He was a very high official in South America. I cannot risk being discovered."

I groaned and dropped my head to the steering wheel.

This kind of drama was repeated whenever we met so that she could pay for services at the vault. In the beginning, while her father was kept in dry ice, the cost was six hundred dollars a month, payable in three-month increments. Laura always paid in cash that she carried in a brown paper bag. She quickly removed the cash from the bag, looking around very carefully to make sure we weren't being watched. It was all so strange that it made me feel as though we were transacting some kind of dope deal. I hurriedly counted the cash and wrote her a receipt; then we talked for about fifteen minutes.

I tried to discover the purpose of all this expense and effort. The only phone number I had was an answering service in New York. When I left messages, she usually called back the next day. I eventually surmised that she wanted her father placed in an upright MVE capsule. She agreed to pay two thousand dollars for each three-month storage-and-maintenance period, plus an additional three thousand dollars toward the purchase of an MVE capsule.

Laura made the first payment of five thousand dollars during a clandestine meeting in Long Beach, in the parking lot of the Hotel Queen Mary. Shortly after I relocated her father into a capsule, she came twice to the vault to see him in the liquid nitrogen. After her second visit, I never heard from Laura again. It was frustrating living in that uncertainty and flux. She had several more payments of five thousand dollars remaining to cover the cost of purchasing and storing her new MVE capsule, and, like so many others, she became delinquent in maintenance charges.

For over a year I left messages threatening to remove her father from the capsule if she did not pay her debt. Fourteen months after receiving only the first five-thousand-dollar payment, I received a letter from a New York attorney claiming that I had not delivered her capsule and demanding a refund of the five thousand dollars. I immediately called him and explained that I had not heard from Laura for over a year. Before I could go any further, he stopped me and explained that he himself had been unable to locate her for going on nine months and was no longer going to represent her.

This was the last dealing I had related to this unusual woman. My conclusion was that she had decided to end her father's cosmetic preservation and this was her unusual method of dealing with his remains. Although I never heard from Laura again, her father remains in the Chatsworth vault to this day.

CHAPTER 12

Vacuum and Vanity

FOR TWO YEARS, GENEVIEVE DE LA POTERIE and Mildred Harrington remained in dry ice—a source of ever-present torture for me, since they needed a less-tenuous, more stable home. Their current accommodation was a four-inch-thick Styrofoam cold-storage box with a one-inch-thick wood exterior. We thought this adequate to hold a human body biologically intact for up to five years, but the dry ice needed to fill the box weekly was prohibitively expensive. I had a solution though. Steven Mandell was in a cryonics capsule, but I couldn't locate his mother and no one was paying for his liquid nitrogen. I didn't want a replay of the first capsule meltdown. I knew I was repeating so many of my earlier actions that had led to failure the first time. Desperate to save all three patients, I decided to open Steven's capsule and place Genevieve's and Mildred's bodies inside with him.

For the first time since I had begun cryonics, I dreamed about death. I had a nightmare that I was laughing and having a great time. Meanwhile I heard a little weak voice say, "Mommy! Daddy! Mr. Bob!" With the feeble voice came the echo of little fists clanging against metal. It was Genevieve crying out for us. She was buried alive, slowly warming and slowly dying. "Mommy! Daddy!" No one had rescued her. I pictured the Grim Reaper sneaking toward her, bringing decay and permanent loss with every inch. The shadow of death was coming closer and closer to her sweet face. I tried to reach her, but I was surrounded by a fog of liquid nitrogen vapor. I felt my way through, but her voice was dissolving into the mist. I finally reached her, finally felt a loose tendril of her hair, and had a momentary flash of relief. Then hideous guilt washed over me as I realized she was no longer Genevieve but rather a crumpled, sad mass that used to be Genevieve.

Breathless, I sat up in my bed and clawed at my covers, whimpering and breathing loud and fast. My bedroom seemed strange now—like it didn't belong to me. Eerie light from the street lamps streamed through the window as Elaine slept beside me. The recesses of my brain could still hear the banging sound inside a metal capsule. I looked around my room, scared and worried about what I might have done and what I hadn't yet accomplished. Genevieve needed me and I couldn't fail her. I would protect her and all my frozen heroes from the shadow of death.

With little funds to continue, my only prayer was to somehow find the money to keep Steven's capsule functioning until help fell from heaven! I looked around me at the cemetery with its vast sea of headstones and felt sure that heaven still existed. Despite the inevitability of death, I wanted to delay it as long as possible. Cryonics for me was about extending life—not about immortality.

After two weeks of preparation, I was a nervous wreck on the day of the patient transfer. With Joseph Klockgether, Frank Farrell, and our trusty welder, Ray Fields, I knew I had an experienced team. I examined the necessary equipment three times: coolers with cold water, four dewars filled with liquid nitrogen, another four empty dewars, gigantic wrenches, Mylar foil, the diamond saw, a welding torch, gloves, lots of dry towels, and a cooler packed with two dozen of my wife's sandwiches, enough to last a long day for four ravenous men. I looked around the heavy-equipment yard at the back of the cemetery grounds; the early morning light still appeared golden. I was glad our enclosure prevented people from seeing our unusual procedure, since I didn't want people interrupting our important work and asking impertinent questions.

Addressing the three men helping me, I said, "Let's discuss this beforehand, because perfection is paramount—no foul-ups. We're performing a heroic undertaking today; we're saving three lives, so let's keep focused on that goal." They nodded in agreement, and I felt satisfied they understood the stakes of our task.

I looked at Ray and said, "This job requires a master craftsman, that's you, to cut off the end of the capsule's inner chamber. We'll take the capsule lid off and transfer Genevieve and Mrs. Harrington into the chamber with Steven. They'll be heavy, and we'll all have to help. Once they're in, we'll reassemble the capsule with . . . absolutely . . . perfect . . . alignment," I staccatoed that phrase, "and re-weld the capsule together. Again, the welding seam needs to be perfect and without breaks so that we'll be able to maintain a perfect vacuum between the two cylinders. *Perfection* is our goal for today—I cannot stress that enough. Any mistakes will be costly and could be catastrophic."

I saw from the wide-eyed, open-mouthed stares of my helpers that they felt overwhelmed. Trying to reassure them I said, "I know it's a huge agenda, but we have no other choice to save all three patients." After I answered a few questions, I did one last equipment check, clapped my hands in excitement, slapped Ray's back, and said, "Let's get going then. We've got a long day ahead."

For two hours we drained the nitrogen. The welder cut a perfect semi-circle around the capsule's end, using a diamond-tipped blade to slice through the stainless steel, and removed the end of the inner capsule. There were no sparks during the cutting, just a loud whirring and a clean break. As we lowered the heavy stainless-steel piece to the ground, the fog-like vapor from the liquid nitrogen dissipated and revealed Steven Mandell's handsome face. The scene was magical, not scary or spooky; he appeared like a prince awaiting an enchanted kiss.

I was prepared for this, but Ray was still unaccustomed to our mission. "How old was he?" Ray asked.

I placed my hand over Steven's. "Five years ago, he was twenty-four."

Without the nitrogen, the exterior of the warmed capsule developed a layer of ice, like a frosted beer mug, and turned everything a ghostly white. Later that frost melted into a thick film of condensation, and we swabbed the capsule with our towels.

Since heat was always our patients' enemy, we hurried as fast as the fifteen-hundred-pound capsule allowed. We had Mildred and Genevieve in a temporary storage container filled with dry ice. We first moved

Mildred; she looked regal in her favorite white wrap dress. Wearing thick gloves, we lifted her from the container and eased her inside the metal capsule. I didn't know why a frozen person felt so heavy, but it took all our strength to move her. After a little positioning, we picked up my beloved Genevieve. She was encased within shiny Mylar foil, and I couldn't see her sweet eyes—chocolate eyes, I remembered. I ran my gloved hand over the Mylar covering her hair and then placed her into the bottom of the capsule next to Mildred.

It took three hours to open up the capsule, another hour to put Genevieve and Mildred in the capsule, four hours to close it, and another hour to align the capsule. Before welding, we covered the interior part of the capsule and the patients with Mylar to minimize their exposure to the heat of the welding. I reiterated that everything had to be done properly.

Watching the intense blue flame as Ray passed his welding torch across the stainless-steel capsule, I was struck by the intense contrasts playing out during our transfer. The welding torch was hotter than the hottest day in the Sahara; the capsule was colder than the coldest night in Siberia. Hot sweat trickled down my face, and cold condensation dripped off the capsule. The heavy capsule was filled with dense bodies and enshrouded by the diaphanous fog of the dry ice.

After the welding, I leaned over to examine the seam, smiled up at Ray, and said, "You did great, truly." Although I wasn't an expert, the weld looked perfect.

We grabbed our half-dozen coolers of cold water and poured them into the inner chamber to quickly cool it. With the capsule now sealed, we bolted on the outer steel lid. The pump needed an hour to reach a good vacuum between the inner and outer cylinders.

The final step was to fill the capsule with liquid nitrogen from the four large dewars. Finally our three patients were sealed and fully supplied with nitrogen. After thanking everyone, I needed to go home and take a much-needed shower and rest.

As I drove out of the cemetery, I checked my watch and realized our task had taken thirteen hours to complete. Hopefully we had guaranteed that our three frozen friends someday would open their eyes and realize they had traveled in the cryonics time machine. Indeed, I felt relieved and optimistic since we had made so much progress.

I returned the next day to see if the welding had been successful. The capsule's performance seemed promising and holding at a tolerable vacuum level, but we needed weeks of observation before I could relax. If it continued performing well, we could lower the capsule into the vault permanently. Only then would I believe these patients were safe.

For the next few months, I monitored the capsule daily and felt forlorn. These initial capsules for human storage were manufactured by Ed Hope, who was a wigmaker, not an engineer, and produced them only to make money. The design was seriously flawed, and the vessel acted like a leaky faucet; everything depended on those vacuum pumps providing the necessary insulation to hold the liquid nitrogen. Our worst problem was the intense heat at Chatsworth during the summer months. The hundred-degree temperatures played havoc with the performance of the pumps.

———

I received a telephone call from Claire Halpert, who lived somewhere in the Southeast. Like Pauline Mandell and Nick DeBlasio, she had contracted with Curtis and the CSNY for freezing services and later gone to battle with them. Her mother, Clara Dostal, had stated in her will that the family could not close their mother's trust until she was frozen and suspended. They had CSNY perform the perfusion and freezing and had her in temporary dry-ice storage.

Clara had set aside money in the trust to pay for everything, including perpetual care. Claire and her brother, Richard, were against having their mother suspended and had other ideas. I didn't know it at the time, but Curtis had sent them to me, telling them that I offered monthly plans for my patients. Mostly he just wanted to get rid of them. In retrospect, I should have followed his model. When the patients' families stopped making payments, Curtis notified them that he was pulling the plug and to retrieve their capsule. He also required the patient's families to purchase their own capsules.

Claire told me over the phone that she did not want to deal with the CSNY and wanted me to transfer her mother to my facility in Chatsworth. God knew I could use one paying customer, but I was disturbed by her tone. She sounded too authoritarian—and also a little wacko. She seemed like she wanted her mother's suspension off her hands. My innards were screaming at me, "Don't do it!" I would have to tread carefully this time.

She wanted me to fly to New York City, check her mother's condition, and arrange to have her flown out to California. I told Claire I needed $2,300 for my travel expenses and shipping arrangements for her mother. I hadn't made any promises at this point. Taking over her mother's suspension was contingent on several factors, including her mother's condition, her willingness to pay for perpetual care, and her attitude. I also wanted Curtis's opinion about the situation.

Claire gave me her brother's phone number and advised me to call Richard once I arrived in New York. He would escort me to the CSNY.

Ten days later, I arrived in New York City and called Curtis Henderson to tell him I was in town at Claire Halpert's request to check out her mother's condition and to possibly arrange her transfer to my facility.

He acted shocked at first but quickly responded, "I hope you're taking this nutcake's mother out of here today!"

"No," I responded slowly, carefully. "I'm just coming out to meet with the son, to examine the capsule, and to learn what the hell is going on with all this craziness."

Curtis sucked in his breath. "You mean you haven't met these people yet?"

"Uh-uh."

"You're in for a surprise. Call me when you're ready to come out, and I'll meet you myself."

After hanging up, dread washed over me. I was anxious to get this meeting done and over with.

That evening I called Richard Dostal from my hotel room.

"Good evening," I started. "This is Bob Nelson from California. Your sister asked me to call you when I got into town to discuss transferring your mom to the CSC's storage facility in California."

After a long silence he answered, "Who the hell are you, and what the hell are you talking about?"

I groaned; that was not the reaction I expected.

"Have you spoken to your sister? She hired me to fly to New York and discuss arrangements to ship your mother to California."

"You know," he responded, sounding cold and unapproachable, "you're as nutty as the rest of them sons-of-bitches. I'll make this as clear as ice water to you, maybe then you'll get it. My mother is dead. Understand? She ain't ever coming back. Not now, not ever. And as soon as her estate is settled, she's going into the ground and be buried, just like she's supposed to. Like normal people do. Do you hear what I'm saying? You body freezers are nuttier than a fuckin' fruit cake. And my sister—she's nuttier than all of you screwballs put together. Do you understand me?"

I gritted my teeth and replied, "Yes, sir, I hear you perfectly."

"Then do me a favor; don't ever call me again. I hate the idea of it." Click.

I flew all the way to New York City for this? I didn't blame him—just his cuckoo sister. I was pissed off, but then I started giggling. I couldn't help myself. I ordered room service and picked the most expensive entree on the menu—filet mignon. I had flown three thousand miles for dinner at a New York hotel, so it should be memorable. Besides, Claire was paying.

I was too embarrassed to call Curtis Henderson, and I felt he didn't want me sniffing around his facility anyway. I didn't bother contacting Claire Halpert either. I didn't need to borrow her troubles.

When I returned to California, there were messages waiting for me at the office from Claire. I ignored her and her demand for her money back. She had wasted my time and subjected me to an unwarranted berating by her brother.

She continued trying to reach me, and I continued ignoring her until I heard she had begun legal action. By that time the money was gone and I had no way of raising it. I contacted her and offered to pay back all but eight hundred dollars in fifty-dollar monthly installments. It was the best I could do. She didn't accept my offer, nor did she decline it. She simply hung up.

CHAPTER 13

Even with Cryonics,
There Is No Escaping Hell

LIFE INTERVENED WITH HORRIFIC TIMING. My brother called and said my mother was in critical condition in Boston City Hospital. My mom's leg was black with gangrene and would kill her within forty-eight hours if the hospital didn't amputate. My brother John refused to give permission without me. I made arrangements with Joe Mendoza, the grounds-keeper at Chatsworth, to look after the capsule and flew to Boston to sign the hospital's papers. Mom's recovery from the operation was remarkable, considering all her problems. She'd had crippling asthma and serious heart problems since childhood. She was also a lifelong smoker and a breast cancer survivor. She had no business being alive at all, but her will was stronger than the hurricane-force winds she'd battled for decades.

At the Boston airport, a fat man came up to me, an inquisitive look shadowing his face. "Isn't your name Buccelli?" That was Big John's name, which I had abandoned years earlier after my stepfather's murder.

I said, "Yes, it . . . is."

He stuck out his hand. "Mine's Sheehy."

His name clicked; this man was the brother of a cherished childhood friend. "Richard!" I yelled. "My God, where is John?" We had lived in the same neighborhood, but I had lost track of him a decade earlier. My long-lost friend now lived in Maine and spent most of his time on his lobster boat. John's life goal had been a lobster-fishing business, and I felt elated to hear he had achieved his dream.

"Richard," I said as the line inched forward to board the plane, "please tell me how to reach him."

"I'm a cop," he answered, "so I can't do that without his permission. Give me your address, and he'll be in touch with you, I promise."

I was thrilled for this chance encounter. What a good trip!

Three days later I received a letter from John. *Dear Bob, am I surprised? Not really; a friendship such as ours was destined to come full circle. Please visit me whenever you can. A pot of lobsters will be waiting for you.*

It was two months before I could get to Maine and hug my old friend. Like he promised, the lobsters were waiting. The evening I arrived, John sat me down and covered my plate with three of them.

When I began to protest, he informed me the Maine record was held by a lumberjack who had devoured twenty-six lobsters at a single sitting. "So shut up and eat!" he ordered.

Thirty minutes later I could not eat another bite. I had eaten six lobsters and was officially declared the West Coast Lobster-Eating Sissy.

After dinner I received a call from Joe Mendoza, the Chatsworth groundskeeper who was watching the capsule for me along with his usual maintenance work.

The pump on the capsule had failed, he said, but had been fixed and all was okay again. Actually the pump had been replaced by our nitrogen supplier. Still, I was worried. I knew this trip was dangerous, since that capsule was functioning on borrowed time.

I flew home to California five days later. During the long flight, I looked out the window at blackness everywhere below, feeling lucky for the rare chance to reflect on our progress. I was soaring from visiting my friend, but the trip reminded me of how much I had sacrificed for the capsule: no vacations, no time that I wasn't free from obligations. The whole world was on my shoulders. I had accomplished so much with the cryonics program, but we had no money to improve the capsules and keep them safe.

I was too sentimental and made bad decisions; I could never say no to my friends because "no" meant I would be killing their future, their hope, and their possibility of a tomorrow. I still believed in hope and possibility, but those lofty concepts didn't matter, since I had created a nightmare of responsibility. I knew CSC would be flourishing if I had not frozen and maintained people who did not make proper financial arrangements. *How could I have let this happen?* There was no one else to blame.

I smiled at a little girl across the aisle. She reminded me of Genevieve; she had the same brown pixie haircut and bounced a Mickey Mouse doll on her tray table, sending my mind back to the wonderful day I had spent with my young friend at Disneyland. What could I do now for Genevieve? It seemed everything I did was never enough. The problems weren't lack of time, devotion, or courage; the problem was money. I remembered my dad's mob friends tossing money around recklessly—a thousand bucks for dinner, another grand for a suit. But for me, money was life and breath and liquid nitrogen.

My primary worry now was that the vacuum leak in the capsule would get worse. Somehow I had to find the money to purchase a better capsule; somehow I had to make it happen. . . .

I drove directly home and fell into bed, exhausted. I spent a few hours the next morning with my family, after not seeing them for two weeks. I made breakfast, giving Elaine a break, and ran lines with Lori for her school play. I was nervous about the capsule. Surely, I thought, since I hadn't heard from Joe again, everything was fine. But the butterflies in my stomach brought a pervasive worry.

I entered the cemetery grounds just after ten o'clock. It was a beautiful morning. The pristine, lush park and the smell of fresh-cut grass transformed my trepidations into optimism as I drove to the capsule at the back of the cemetery. The sunshine altered my mood. But when I approached the yard, I noticed an eerie silence when I turned off the car engine. At first I couldn't identify what was different. Hideous realization washed over me; the vacuum pump was not running!

I stood there for a few minutes in stunned disbelief before sprinting up to the capsule. I studied the vent pipe, knowing it should have a slight fog from the evaporating liquid nitrogen. I saw nothing.

I paced around the capsule for several minutes, trying to muster the courage to touch the vent. If it was cold then things were okay. But if it wasn't . . . I could not bear even to think about it! My mind tumbled over the consequences if it felt warm, imagining scenes of distraught families screaming and crying that I had failed them. If the vent was warm, my entire life would come crashing down on me.

Five minutes passed before I finally touched the vent. The vent was not just warm. *It was hot!* That heat penetrated straight to my heart and singed my soul. How long had it been this way? Then Genevieve's face appeared in my mind. The thought of her decaying deep inside this fifteen-hundred-pound pressure cooker drove me to my knees, and I cried. I cried harder and longer than ever before, until my face was wet from the flow of tears and snot, and my chest pained from relentless heaving. The meticulously manicured cemetery grass beneath me was a green blur, and in that blur I saw the faces of those lost after so much passion and effort expended to save them.

After what seemed like a very long time, I stood back up on wobbly legs. My emotions rapidly passed from devastation and despair to anger, and then to rage. *What the fuck happened?* I had to find Joe. I would tear him apart! I would . . . no. I could do nothing to him. He was not an engineer; he was a groundskeeper. I chose him to look after things. This catastrophe was my fault, not his.

As I careened around the winding roads like I was escaping hell, people attending funerals all turned toward me. I sped through the park looking for Joe, and I finally found him fixing a sprinkler on the north end of the grounds. I pulled up and I could see his face turn beet-red as I approached. He knew I was pissed.

I screamed, "Joe, what in the hell happened!"

"Well," he said in a thick accent, "several days ago after I call you I see the pump, she's a-stop again, so I call the number you give me. I tell them three times; they say what? what? I'm tell them, come, come. They never come. I don't know what to do."

"Why didn't you call me?" I fumed.

"I don-a know. I call them. They don-a come back."

Still livid, I shoved him toward the sprinkler and got him wet, but then I calmed down. Yelling at him accomplished nothing. I turned around, disgusted, and walked away. I barged into the cemetery office, parked myself at Joe's desk, and jerked the rotary dial on the telephone as I spun each number to call Gilmore Liquid Air. "I made full arrangements for your company to come to Chatsworth and deal with emergencies. We called with an emergency and nobody came." I was yelling but didn't care. "Do you know the consequences—the ramifications—of this?"

"Please hold." The singsong reply of the operator made me more upset. A minute later I was talking to the owner of the company, Mrs. Gilmore herself.

Trying not to cry, I again explained what happened.

The owner's response was measured but sympathetic. "We received a call from someone who couldn't speak English very well. He kept saying something about fixing a pump. I finally spoke to him and told him we didn't fix pumps. Then he just kept repeating himself over and over; he finally hung up. I had no idea he was talking about cryonics or had any connection with your company."

Well there it was—the dumbest explanation ever given for condemning three human beings. I had made all the arrangements, hired all the actors, and directed the entire scenario. Yet I failed to consider that the man I had charged with looking after the heart of the operation barely spoke English. I was solely responsible for the death of these three lost friends. We had tried so hard, but I had failed them even though I had spent so much time, energy, and money.

All for nothing.

Dropping into Joe's office chair, I had to figure out a plan. I called Gilmore back and asked them to deliver liquid nitrogen to the capsule site. I knew it was useless to keep feeding nitrogen into the capsule. The damage was done. They were dead—not just clinically dead but irrevocably gone—killed by my mistakes and the California sun. I needed time to think about the events that had created this tragedy.

I returned to the vault, hoping for some altered reality. I placed a tentative finger on the vent pipe; it was hot of course. I sank to the earth and sat on the ground. The entire day, my body was splayed against the sweltering-hot stainless steel of the outer capsule. I couldn't move from the scorching metal. I considered it penance—my punishment for failing my three patients. I wanted to share their fate; the waning sun spared me, but not them.

After several hours I allowed myself the undeserved luxury of standing up and stretching. I wished I hadn't, for I saw the dark shadow of the surrounding fence creeping slowly across the capsule, inexorably shrouding its inhabitants in darkness. The shadow of death that I had always feared came that day. For years I had stood ready to do battle with the Grim Reaper, poised with dry ice and liquid nitrogen instead of a cold steel sword. My failure was irrevocable and absolute.

In the late afternoon, a delivery truck from Gilmore arrived with more nitrogen. I poured the liquid nitrogen into the capsule; the backsplash felt like hundreds of tiny needles on my arm. Finally I was relieved to see the capsule's shroud of fog; I trudged to my car to head home.

My daughters tackled me with hugs when I arrived. Elaine saw my beaten face, noticed me wince, and sent the girls off to watch television. This amazing woman who knew me so well knew instantly that my world had somehow crumbled.

During many of our relationship's dramatic moments, she had been the one crying or about to cry; now it was my turn. She grabbed a bottle of aloe and smeared it onto the burns where I'd pressed against the hot metal.

"I lost them. They're gone." I said. We didn't speak again that night, she just held me in her arms, smoothed my hair, and tried with love to ease the pain.

After a week of dwelling on the capsule loss, I knew I had to inform the families directly. If their relatives wanted to beat me up, then so be it. Remembering all the thrashings from my childhood, I figured this probably would be the first one I truly deserved.

It was now 1974, the better part of a decade since I had taken the reins with such lofty dreams, guiding CSC toward developing facilities for cryonic suspension. Now I confronted the most god-awful task of my entire life. I must tell Guy de la Poterie that I had failed to keep his daughter safe and preserved. After all his effort and mine, his daughter's capsule failed when I was far away visiting my friend.

I also needed to face Mildred's sons and inform them of their mother's loss in the same capsule. I had lost touch with Pauline Mandell, Steven's mother, and didn't know how to contact her.

I called Guy from my mom's home in Boston before I left for Montreal to confirm our visit.

He agreed to meet me at the airport but asked, "Why the sudden visit?"

I avoided answering, asking instead, "Can we meet for coffee?"

"A cup of coffee? You're always telling me how tight money is, and now you want to fly to Montreal for a cup of coffee?" I could hear the panic in his voice as his French accent grew stronger. "What's happening with my Genevieve?"

He sounded frantic, but I still didn't want to answer. I looked around my mom's house. It felt strange being here and being yelled at. I was a kid again—a twelve-year-old screw-up.

I couldn't stall any longer, making him wait and worry just so that my confession could match the script I had played out in my mind.

There was such agony in my heart as I cleared my throat and shakily began. I told him about my trip and how the capsule had failed while I was away. "I had made arrangements for the capsule, but it still happened. The responsibility is mine."

Guy listened silently; then after a long pause he asked, "How long was the capsule without liquid nitrogen?"

"My best guess is five days. I am so sorry, Guy."

I waited in silence for a few minutes before Guy asked, "Does the capsule have liquid nitrogen now?"

"Yes, I refilled it, and it's being checked daily by my assistant Frank Farrell."

"Well that's good," he said. "I guess there is nothing we can do but continue storing her."

It was a reaction I had not anticipated. Several days of decomposition seemed like an eternity. Numb with disbelief but not wanting to inflict additional pain, I cowardly replied, "I'll do that if it's what you want."

After this brief conversation, Guy said he was not feeling well and hung up.

I was tempted to call Guy back and fully explain the ramifications of the capsule failure, but I never did—and I never went to Canada.

My next stop was cold and rainy Des Moines, Iowa. Terry Harrington was standing by the gate with a masculine-looking woman. She was dressed all in black, carrying a black umbrella and clutching Terry's arm. We went to a nearby restaurant, and Terry introduced her as his wife. Now I felt sure I'd entered some alternate reality. The last time I saw Terry and his brother, I felt convinced they were gay, and now he was married.

I raised my eyebrows and shook my head, but I needed to focus on my difficult task of telling Terry the truth. His brother, Dennis, didn't meet us, and I felt less stressed facing Terry since I had already spoken to Guy. I told Terry that the capsule had failed for several days. To my surprise he did not appear at all upset. Like Guy, he did not realize the consequences of that capsule failure.

He repeated what Guy had said. "I guess the only thing we can do is fill it up and keep on going."

I sat there stunned, my coffee cup poised in midair. Years earlier I had carefully educated both Guy and the Harrington brothers about cryonics, yet both seemed completely unfazed by those days of soaring temperatures. I opened my mouth to object, but again I took the coward's way and didn't correct his assumptions.

Without much more to say, our meeting quickly ended. I flew to Michigan, where Professor Ettinger met me in the waiting area at the Detroit airport. We sat down in the lounge, and I told him about the capsule failure.

He was saddened by the news, but he had always been a wise, incredibly perceptive man. He patted my hand. "Disappointments on our path are the price we sometimes pay for success." He was reassuring and offered his condolences.

I couldn't let it go that easily. "All my grand ideas and lofty goals, all the excitement from those early heady days reduced to this. . . . Everything seems impossible now."

My voice trailed off. I hated this realization, because I had begun this journey with such overwhelming certainty. All those early hopes, those early feelings that I was creating a monumental shift in humanity, had been reduced to this capsule failure—my utter failure. That shift—that death of a dream—was just as painful as the death of these three people. I couldn't acknowledge the death of my dream. I had to persevere.

Professor Ettinger put his arm over my shoulder. "The purpose of life is to discover the purpose of life. This is a tragedy, but a bigger tragedy would be if you lost your faith."

I melted into an embrace and stayed like that for a long while, just rocking back and forth on the airport couch. He understood my heartbreak and held me for a long time. With him I didn't have to be strong or the man with all the answers. He truly was the father I had always needed. Eventually I pulled back and steeled myself to say good-bye to this wonderful man.

I arrived home in California thoroughly confused. *What had just happened?* To know what to do next, I had to understand the reactions of Guy de la Poterie and Terry Harrington.

My far-fetched conclusion was that there might be some hope left for those in the capsule. Although neither my heart nor my mind could believe it, I decided to keep the capsule operating for as long I could manage.

And so began three more years of filling the capsule with liquid nitrogen. I rarely dwelled on the one-week failure and certainly never mentioned it to other CSC members; I had learned well from the Mafia not to tell people more than necessary. During that time I spent thousands of dollars of my own money on my fool's errand—I knew the one week at hot temperatures had ended everything for my three heroes. It was the most basic lesson of low-temperature biology.

One day in early October 1974, I was at the CSC office in Santa Monica when I received a phone call from Tom Porter. His six-year-old son Sam was dying of leukemia, and he wanted to discuss placing him in suspension. I scheduled a meeting for nine the next morning at Klockgether's mortuary. When I arrived and introduced myself, Tom explained that doctors had given his son a week or two.

Tom had investigated cryonics and wanted to obtain information about storing his son's capsule at the Chatsworth vault. He had already purchased a new upright capsule manufactured by Andonian Cryogenics, a competitor of MVE. I did a quick calculation in my head; the capsule would fit inside the vault with its lid one foot below the ceiling. All he needed was a safe, legal place to store, service, and monitor his son's capsule.

Tom had gray hair and was very overweight, probably from overworking and dealing with his son's illness. I agreed to meet him later that week to finalize our deal. He was an assistant district attorney, and since he already had a capsule, those two factors increased my confidence that he would keep his word and not disappoint me like so many had before. I tried asking him about his son Sam, but Tom merely described him as a sweet boy. Although quite articulate, Tom never divulged his personal turmoil.

He promised he would make all arrangements and payments to fill the capsule with liquid nitrogen each month. He also wanted to monitor all the steps of safe storage and maintenance. He trusted no one else. "The perfusion, capsule space, and security will cost ten thousand dollars, and that's on top of the monthly liquid nitrogen replacement." I paused and breathed loudly for emphasis. "However, if you allow another person in that capsule with your son, I'll do it for three thousand dollars."

He didn't hesitate. He reached into his pocket, pulled out a wad of cash, counted off three thousand dollars, and asked, "When can I have the capsule delivered?"

I thumbed the bills and answered, "In two days."

"Would 1:00 p.m. be okay?"

I agreed but was somewhat taken aback by the speed at which all this was transpiring. "Tom, you sure don't waste time."

"I can't afford to," he answered. "Between my job and my son being so close to death, time is invaluable to me."

It bothered me that there was no documentation of these decisions, but Tom wanted no paperwork; he didn't want any word of his son's cryonic suspension getting out. He knew that his extended family would have had fierce objections. I figured an assistant DA would want a record of his agreements, but this one didn't.

I was waiting at the vault on Thursday when the new upright capsule arrived, accompanied by a crane. I couldn't resist touching the shiny metallic container; it already felt hot from the sun's radiation, and I was amazed again at the temperature drop between the inside and outside of the cylinder—a 400°F difference across six inches. If I had had something like this capsule for my other patients, they would still have been with us.

Afterwards we developed a mutual trust, and he allowed me to monitor the liquid nitrogen delivery for him. Tom was dependable and always did exactly what he promised.

About a week later, on October 11, his little son passed away. After Joseph Klockgether completed the perfusion, the boy was placed into the stainless-steel capsule to await the future. Over the next three years, Tom and his wife came out several times to visit their son. And as Tom had promised, he was at the cemetery each month when the liquid nitrogen truck arrived.

On two occasions they wanted to open the capsule and view their son. Although I didn't want to intrude on such intensely personal moments, it amazed me to see how much it meant to Tom and his wife to see their son as he appeared when he died—still young and still very much their little boy. The nitrogen hadn't been refilled yet that day, so the liquid level was low enough that they could touch Sam's cold face. His wife reached into the capsule with a tentative hand and fingered her precious son's hair. She continued for several minutes, biting her lip to ward off tears. I could tell that the memories overwhelmed her. She brought back her hand as though the cold capsule had turned hot, and she buried her face into Tom's shoulder to muffle her crying.

I had been involved with cryonics for many years, almost a decade at that point, and had been witness to some of the most tumultuous moments in people's lives. However, I realized that cryonics provided another benefit over normal burial techniques. When a person, especially a child, dies, there are so many emotions with the first fiery flood of grief, but also so many responsibilities with the funeral and arrangements. With burial or cremation, those horrific and hectic days are the only opportunity for parents to see their child for the last time before that chance is gone forever. With cryonics, that final good-bye, that last moment of seeing their child, is delayed into the future, when parents are better able to cope with the tragedy of their child's death. As difficult as it was for Tom and his wife to see their son, I watched the profound comfort they gained from the two visits.

—◆—

I had received no money from Pauline Mandell or the Harrington brothers. Occasionally Guy de la Poterie sent me fifty or a hundred dollars. The vault was no longer a joy or my great legacy; instead it was an untenable burden pushing me into early residence at the Chatsworth cemetery. I had run out of money, energy, and the expectation that the CSC could be saved. Once I lost the hope of some guardian angel or miraculous benefactor coming to our aid, I caved. The battle was over, and I could carry the load no longer. I had nothing more to offer the cryonics program.

Three years after the capsule failure, I wrote Guy de la Poterie, explaining that due to the constantly failing capsule, lack of funds, along with my own physical and mental state, I was unable to continue. My wife had divorced me since the capsule failure, and I had neglected my children. I wrote a similar letter to the Harrington brothers. For several years I had been unable to contact Pauline Mandell, so I did not write to her.

I was broken and impoverished. Starting life over again was like climbing a mountain as a sick and naked man. Somehow, I thought, I would survive. It was late fall in 1977, and I still worked as a big-screen repairman. Almost half my salary had gone into the vault.

In that moment I felt like Sisyphus, the mythological Greek king who was punished with the task of forever rolling a rock up a steep hill, only to watch it roll back down and then have to repeat the procedure forever. *Was I guilty of hubris or of too-great optimism? What was my fatal flaw?*

I had taken my last step in my walk across the desert. I was barely a step away from my own demise. I had to let go, but my heart kept screaming, *No! No! Don't let go; hold on just a little longer.* I could not, and as my hand slipped from the vault handle, I wept my final tear and braced myself for my life yet to come.

CHAPTER 14

The End of the Dream

I INFORMED TOM PORTER THAT I WAS RESIGNING as custodian of the vault but assured him that he could continue his son's suspension for as long as he wanted and gave him the keys to the vault. I expected him to move the capsule to another facility or hire someone to monitor it. Much to my surprise, although the capsule was functional and in good condition, Tom decided to end his son's suspension after about a year of servicing it himself. His Catholic parents had religious objections, and he was worried about appearing to be custodian of the Chatsworth vault.

Around March 1979 I cut open the Mandell capsule. Joseph Klockgether removed both children from their capsules as their parents had requested and delivered them to his mortuary for a service and conventional burial in Orange County. Mildred Harrington, Steven Mandell, and Pedro Ladesma were also removed and placed in conventional metal boxes called Ziegler cases. Louis Nisco, Marie Sweet, Russ Stanley, and Helen Kline were left sealed in their capsule. Several years back the Harrington brothers had their father disinterred a year after he was buried and shipped to Chatsworth to be with their mother. Terry had wanted his father to be cryonically suspended, but Joseph and I refused. What would be the point? He remained in his original coffin. They still reside in the Chatsworth vault today, lined up side by side but simply interred like every other resident at the cemetery, their story sadly over.

It was rumored later that the maintenance of Tom's son had been irregular, with one or more episodes of thawing that left visible signs of damage; however, that was definitely untrue. As reliable as an atomic clock, Tom Porter never once was late with a capsule fill. The young boy's service was held at the Rennaker Mortuary, and Joseph Klockgether said he looked perfect. I suspect there might have been some cracking of the skin caused by his direct and sudden placement into the liquid nitrogen. Back in those early days, we did not have the capability to bring the body temperature down to -320°F over a two-day period, as we do today.

I don't believe that Tom Porter or Genevieve's dad, Guy de la Poterie, blamed me personally for the capsule failure and the facility's closure. However, they were bitterly disappointed, and I am sure they felt little goodwill toward me. They had nothing to say to me. They had lost their children twice. Seeing their compounded heartache was one of the saddest experiences of my life.

Just as the vault was closing, my day of reckoning had arrived. The repercussions of my soft heart, bad decisions, and resulting mismanagement hit me like freight train. I had been such a fool, but I had no one to blame but myself.

With cryonics, I had aimed high and flown high, believing that the wonder of preserved life was within my grasp. I wanted to be like the Wright Brothers and became Icarus instead. And like Icarus, I fell hard and far.

I thought that my last time at the vault was the bottom and nothing could be worse. But soon I learned there was always room for more grief when you're on the wrong path.

My friend and the best helper to all cryonics believers, Joseph Klockgether, had malpractice insurance protecting his mortuary business. It was a delicious deep pocket, an invitation to those who loved money. My fear of a brewing monster tornado was well founded.

———

After I shut down the vault, I worked full-time as a technician for RCA as a big-screen repairman. For a while I felt happily lost in boring normalcy and domesticity. That changed when Joseph called me one rainy day.

"Hi, Bob. I've got some bad news. We're getting sued."

"Sued? By whom? For what?"

"The Halperts—"

"Oh, them." I breathed easier; we hadn't done anything for them, and their case wouldn't get any traction.

Ironically, the Halpert family had initiated a complaint against Joseph Klockgether and me for *not* taking control of their mother's storage and maintenance at the CSC vault. We had never met any of the family and had nothing to do with the freezing and storage of their mother.

Joseph had never heard of the Halperts. He had nothing to do with CSNY, the Halperts, or my trip to New York City; but he had malpractice insurance, and that made him a target.

"We're getting sued for *not* transferring a body from CSNY to your facility," he said. "I'd never heard of them."

"Joe, I'm so sorry. I dragged you into this, but this is beyond bizarre. I can't believe they can sue me, let alone you. They'll get tossed out."

"That's not all. Their lawyer found the Harrington brothers and Marie Brown. They're suing for breach of contract, fraud, and everything else their lawyers can imagine."

This stung. I had thought of the Harrington brothers as friends, and I had helped Marie Brown when Ed Hope intended to throw her father's capsule into the street.

"This is all my fault, but don't worry, Joe. It'll be annoying as hell, but we're protected."

He answered, "Yeah, yeah," like he knew that's what I'd say.

I was shocked, yet I knew if people could get money by suing, they would sue. Everything we had done was in good faith, with a clear conscience, and protected under the Anatomical Gift Act.

My friend and attorney, Stella Gramer, assured me that no justifiable legal actions could be taken against me or anyone acting on the society's behalf. Cryonics organizations throughout the country had long operated under the AGA and still do, just like medical institutions that perform dissections and intentional destruction of donated bodies in their students' gross anatomy classes.

That the lawyers put Joseph in their crosshairs was completely unfair. Joseph had donated all of his time to the CSC, but that made no difference.

I learned that they were looking for me to serve a subpoena. Their strategy was to portray me as a despicable con man with Joseph as my cover and to argue that together we had swindled fortunes from our victims.

I decided not to make it easy for the sharks to find me, and I was successful for about a year. However, one day a process server somehow got into my high-security apartment building and knocked on my door. I looked through the peephole and did not respond, so he slid the subpoena under the door.

I didn't have to accept it, but I needed to end my self-imposed house arrest and deal with the legal farce. The document sickened me. It accused me of every god-awful imaginable thing, including swindling many people out of their life savings. I was ordered to give a deposition; I needed help, but I didn't have the money for an attorney.

The plaintiffs' lawyer, Michael Worthington, revolted me at our first deposition. He wasn't focused on the complaining party, the Halperts. Even someone as wormy as Worthington realized he wouldn't have a chance at trial, since we had done nothing for the Halperts, and Joseph had never even heard of them. The lawyer had researched all our patients and found the mother lode with the Harrington brothers, making them the star witnesses. Now he wanted $2.5 million for breach of contract and $10 million in punitive damages.

I answered hundreds of questions as honestly as I could, but with each impertinent question from that snide man, my stomach just felt more nauseated. All I could focus on was his appearance—skinny, hunched over, and swallowed up by his oversize suit. When the deposition was over, Worthington offered to settle the lawsuit for thirty thousand dollars. That sounded like a good deal, but Joseph's insurance company refused, saying the whole case was so absurd it would be laughed out of court. Two weeks later I informed Worthington that the insurance company had rejected his offer.

After returning home from work one night that summer, I caught a report by the Los Angeles CBS affiliate, *Channel 2 News*, with news anchor Peter Pepper: "A big story is just now breaking in Chatsworth,

California, at the Oakwood Memorial Park. A cryonics storage vault containing a huge number of frozen bodies has been abandoned, and all the bodies have been left to rot in an abandoned, filthy, snake-riddled and fly-infested burial vault. The president, Robert Nelson, has absconded with a large fortune meant to care for the perpetual maintenance of the frozen bodies. Nelson is nowhere to be found."

I almost fell off my chair, dumbfounded at this slanderous story. I had never felt so naked and exposed. I worried about my kids; they wouldn't believe it, but they'd have to deal with questions and taunts from their classmates.

I grabbed the phone and called *Channel 2 News*. I told them who I was and demanded to speak to Pepper. After about a ten-minute wait, he came on the line.

"Are you stupid or just nuts?" I asked. I was in no mood to be subtle or polite. "Where the hell did you get that disgustingly untrue story, and why in the world did you not check into the truth of it first?"

Unabashed and with no apparent concern for journalistic ethics, he replied that he went to the facility, broke the lock, and looked inside with his cameras.

"You broke the lock?" I asked, amazed he'd so casually admit to a crime. "And what did you find?"

"Well I, I, don't really know. It looked pretty messy down there!"

I sat there stunned. How could a guy like this Pepper be a news anchor where he could influence millions? "If you're going to run a story, why don't you first listen to the truth?"

"Okay," he said. "When can you be here? Can I interview you about that cryonics vault?"

His offer calmed me down a bit. Hoping I could fix this right now, I said, "I'll come this very moment."

We agreed to meet at two o'clock the next day at the CBS studio in the San Fernando Valley. Exactly at two, I stormed into the studio to rebut their story and to remind Peter Pepper that CBS had committed a felony by breaking and entering a consecrated burial vault. A gorgeous intern ushered me into a large conference room.

Five minutes later Peter Pepper came in, shook my hand, and commented, "I must say I was surprised you'd want an interview. Do you mind if we record you?" Two cameramen entered the room behind him.

I shrugged. "Not at all; I have nothing to hide. As long as you proceed truthfully, I will answer honestly as well."

He gave his opening bit and then turned the camera on me. I began with, "Peter, you got it all wrong. Why were you so devious—breaking into the CSC storage vault and pointing your cameras looking for something? Why didn't you simply discuss it with me, the president of CSC, before you took this illegal action?"

Yes, I was really ex-president by then, but people on the outside knew me as president, so I let it go at that.

Ignoring my charge that he had committed a felony when he broke into our cryonics vault, he responded by asking me another question: "What happened to the enormous trust fund that these patients left you to provide for their perpetual care and preservation?"

"There is no such fund." I banged my fist on the table for emphasis. "Most of them were penniless; no one had a trust fund. Those are lies. When you were at the vault, did your cameraman focus in on some flies that were aboveground, trying to insinuate there were flies inside the vault? Flies could not live inside the vault. Why would you fabricate such a story?"

Pepper looked back at his cameramen and glowered when he saw one smirking. He was used to people fawning over him, not scolding him. He responded by asking me another question: "Where are the hundreds of thousands of dollars that are missing from these people's trust funds?"

"There is no missing money and certainly not hundreds of thousands of dollars." I explained that we had run out of money and could not continue to service the cryogenic capsules without funds. All my years of TV interviews served me well; I could appear calm and look respectable on camera. Pepper paused to smooth his hair and to check his teeth and his suit. Finally satisfied, he continued, "So your organization ran out of money. Did you sometimes rob Peter to pay Paul?"

I responded, "I guess there were times that you could say that."

"Ah ha," he said. "So the question becomes who was 'Peter' and who was 'Paul'?"

I shrugged. "I just did what was necessary to give all my patients a chance to continue on. I spent years fighting for them."

Pepper grimaced and thumped his pencil, disappointed that the story did not have the teeth he wanted.

As I walked out of the CBS studio that afternoon, I discovered the source of the story. Worthington was hiding behind the exit door, and as I left the building, he popped out and handed me another subpoena, which Pepper's cameras caught on film. In reality, Worthington could not serve me a subpoena; he was the plaintiffs' attorney of record, and I had already been served. This was a dummy, serving only for news drama.

I ripped up the phony subpoena as soon as I left the building and was able to breathe fresh air. *Worthington!* I spat out his name. Of course he had engineered the news story. I wanted to boil and butter that snake.

This so-called breaking story was on the news again that night. My "Peter and Paul" statement and the arranged confrontation with Worthington were broadcast, but that was all. Pepper reported that research was ongoing and he would have more at a later date.

Disgusted at Peter Pepper, I called him the next day and said, "Do you realize Worthington made a fool out of you? He used you and he used your news station just to gain publicity for his deep-pockets trial case." I reiterated, "CSC had frozen most of the patients free of charge. Out of the kindness of our hearts, we were trying to get these people into long-term storage."

"How much money did you get to save these frozen bodies of people you have never met?"

"CSC didn't get money, and we had to end the vault; that's the story!"

Pepper had two more questions: "First, how much money did you collect from society members for the maintenance of these frozen patients?"

I answered, "On my soul, not a penny ever from anyone."

"Second," he asked, "what can you tell me about the lawsuit?"

I said, "We have a mortician who often assisted with our cryonics patients. He has malpractice insurance—in other words, deep pockets that Worthington wants to pillage."

After that phone conversation, *Channel 2 News* never again mentioned this sordid fabrication. The cemetery owner, Frank Enderle, considered filing both criminal and civil action against the news station for breaking, entering, and trespassing. Because a crippling stroke rendered him unable to walk or speak, the CBS affiliate managed to avoid legal action.

The next few months were a nightmare of expense and confusion. After the *Channel 2 News* farce, the plaintiffs' attorney, Worthington, inundated me with hundreds of hours of interrogatories, all of which required an attorney.

The pressure continued when a journalist wrote an article about Chatsworth claiming that "the stench near the crypt is disarming, strips away all defenses, spins the stomach into a thousand dizzying somersaults." This was untrue of course. The bodies were placed in sealed containers, wrapped, and intact.

I was tempted to not appear. I would've then lost by default and could simply bankrupt away the judgment. However, I couldn't desert Joseph Klockgether. This money-grabbing scam was an assault not only against me but also against cryonics. Somehow I had to stand by Joseph and fight for justice. I needed a good, but cheap, attorney.

I called the Orange County Legal Aid Society, and they gave me an address and an appointment. When I arrived for my free fifteen-minute consultation, there were twenty other poor people in the waiting room who needed help for their problems. I brought a thirty-pound box filled with years of cryonics documents, Worthington's interrogatories, records, and related evidence. Where the hell could I begin this insane story, with only fifteen minutes to explain everything?

Finally I was called into this tiny cubicle with no room for my box, so the attorney asked me to simply tell him my problem, no records. I began talking ninety miles an hour: "I froze the first man and people started dying, they didn't have any money but I froze them anyway, then the capsules kept failing, then . . ."

By this point, I couldn't understand myself! But I forged ahead. "This little girl I fell in love with, I mean I didn't really fall in love, I just loved her like a daughter. She died and the family didn't have any money but I froze her. I couldn't help myself; she was such a sweetheart. I . . . I . . . I . . ."

"Wait a minute," said the questioner; his name was Winterbotham. "What the hell are you talking about?"

"Cryonics. I'm the ex-president of the Cryonics Society," I explained.

"You mean the organization that puts people in suspended animation?"

Hearing him say *suspended animation* gave me my first glimmer of hope. "Yes," I said. "That's me. I'm being sued. Can you help me?"

He reached into his pocket, took out his card, and gave it to me. "Call me tomorrow after 10:00 a.m." That was against the rules, as he was only supposed to dispense brief legal advice, but he was interested in my story.

I called at ten sharp and made an appointment to meet at his home at 2:00 p.m. We talked for more than four hours, and he reviewed countless documents. This man seemed like the perfect person to combat the sneaky Worthington. He was intelligent and charismatic, and he had a genuine smile. I knew he'd convince a jury to see the truth.

"This case is the most ridiculous effort to extract money from an insurance company I've ever heard," he said. "There's no doubt we'll win the case. I'll just need fifteen thousand dollars to get started."

I accepted and turned over a ton of overdue interrogatories. I gave him a postdated check for three thousand dollars and promised to have the remaining twelve thousand paid within thirty days.

Attorney Winterbotham declared that, with the signed Anatomical Gift Act documents, we could not lose. Although we had all the signed documentation showing donation of body and funds, the Harrington brothers claimed we had made a verbal contract that I would provide a twenty-thousand-dollar MVE capsule and that I would replace the liquid nitrogen forever. That was ludicrous, stupid, and, well, creative fibbing.

The truth was, as I explained, they had said that ten thousand dollars was all they could afford. And the brothers had never made one donation toward their mother's liquid nitrogen cost.

I will always remember his parting words that day: "The fraud is being perpetrated *against* Mr. Klockgether and you, not the other way around."

So now I had a clever attorney who was skilled at preparing a case. All I had to do was come up with another twelve thousand dollars. There was only one way—I had to sell my beloved Porsche Speedster. It was twenty-five years old and the last thing in the world I owned of any value. I had held on to the Porsche through all the hardship, sacrifice, and lean years. During those times, I think I knew in my gut to hang on to the car because I would need that money in my darkest hour. That moment had now come. I had given my word to fight this witch hunt to the end, so that's what I was going to do.

CHAPTER 15

The Trial*

As THE TRIAL BEGAN, Winterbotham and I agreed to alternate driving into Los Angeles each day. This would give us an hour each way to dissect the day's proceedings. He had no set strategy; he planned to refute their lies with the truth. He couldn't understand how their case could prevail once we introduced the Anatomical Gift Act. That sounded wonderful, and it would likely end the argument. I felt confident, mostly.

That first day we arrived at the courthouse on a crisp April morning, it was a circus. Cameramen and reporters shouted questions such as, "How many millions did you rip off, Mr. Nelson?" "Did you ever really freeze anyone?"

Holding my head high, I ignored them and strolled up the concrete steps. I had seen comparable dramas with other defendants play out on television, including my stepfather, Big John. The courtroom loomed before me. I always had needed to be in control, and it was scary to realize I had ceded my fate to the judge, jury, and my lawyer.

"All rise." The bailiff's voice commanded silence, and everyone was settled.

The jury box was on the extreme left of the courtroom, opposite a bank of windows and an evidence table that spanned the length of the courtroom. Klockgether, our attorneys, and I sat on the right side of the aisle, farthest from the jury. From the statue of Blind Justice to the

---

* This chapter, which deals with the cryonics trial of 1981, is a reconstruction from my memory of the proceedings and is not offered as verbatim testimony.

imposing mahogany throne for the judge, everything seemed so grand and imperious. Judge Shelby was big too; the zipper on his black robe was battling with his roly-poly belly. With his girth and white beard, I hoped he'd begin court by saying "Ho, ho, ho" and offer to bring me a "not guilty" verdict for Christmas. When the court session began, the jury selection was a tug-of-war between the plaintiffs and us. They wanted older, conservative people; we wanted the fresh-faced young folks and no grumps.

My first surprise was Thomas Nothern, newly installed cocounsel to the plaintiff, and I realized my case had just become a lot harder. I had envisioned the slimy, devious Worthington repulsing the jury. In contrast, Nothern was so charming he seemed destined for a courtroom. He was a slight man with a severely deformed left leg, so he walked with crutches. He was good-looking and soft-spoken, and with his light Southern drawl, he appeared a kind and friendly gentleman.

As Nothern approached the jury box for his opening statement, he introduced Worthington, the Harrington brothers, and their witnesses. Nothern then explained to the jury how his clients had been duped and defrauded out of thirty-five thousand dollars. He told them that I had come to Des Moines, Iowa, and froze their mother, shipped her to California, put her in temporary dry-ice storage, and then stole their ten thousand dollars, which they said was their mother's entire bequest.

The Harringtons claimed that I promised to provide their mom with a new twenty-thousand-dollar MVE capsule and that I would pay for the liquid nitrogen until their mother could be brought back to life. No matter how long it took! Although they acknowledged they had given only ten thousand dollars to CSC, they wanted an additional fifteen thousand dollars, which they had supposedly spent for her memorial service two years after she had died.

Also, they wanted another ten thousand dollars because their father, who had never been frozen, had been disinterred a year after his death and shipped to Chatsworth to reside with their mother. They claimed I had told them that the CSC had plenty of funds and didn't need any help paying for liquid nitrogen or maintenance. My attorney had his nose in his yellow legal pad, scribbling down notes. It worried me, though, that his hand trembled as his pen flew across the page. He had told me he was confident about our chances, and now he was acting nervous.

When Nothern spoke, he captivated people in an almost magical way. I couldn't help but like him; even more important, I couldn't help but believe him.

"This was a *fraud*," Nothern intoned, his palms resting on the railing of the jury box, "perpetrated on the country and the world. Bob Nelson was the 'General,' the leader who deceived people in their *grief,* when they were ready to grasp at any straw to save or bring back a loved one from death. Yes, ladies and gentlemen, it was all just a *scam,* designed to rip people off for their money during the most tragic and vulnerable moment of their life."

I wanted to scream. *If that was true, why was the CSC vault full of people who paid nothing to get frozen?* Nothern's opening statement was powerful, and he made it so damn believable. I battled my feelings of sympathy for him as he struggled to return to the plaintiff's table on his crutches.

It was now Winterbotham's turn to address the jury. My attorney began by asking them to use plain common sense. "Does it seem even remotely possible that my client, Mr. Nelson, would say, 'Give CSC ten thousand dollars and we will give you a state-of-the-art MVE capsule that cannot be purchased anywhere in the world for less than twenty thousand dollars'? Does it make sense that CSC, an experimental research society that exists solely on donations, would also perform a complete perfusion and cryogenic freezing on the plaintiffs' mother in Iowa? That CSC would pay all the plane fares round-trip for my client and Joseph Klockgether? Then they would ship the plaintiffs' mother to California and place her in temporary storage for maybe two years, after which they would put her into a capsule and my client would pay the monthly replacement cost of liquid nitrogen to her capsule forever?"

Winterbotham stopped to gauge his effectiveness. "The plaintiffs' argument is silly, and it is easy to show that CSC never agreed to any such nonsense. Both brothers signed the contract that shows the substance of the real agreement made that day. CSC has always expressed in its publications and television and radio appearances that the cost of a complete cryonic suspension was ten thousand dollars plus adequate funds invested to create an endowment for liquid nitrogen replacement, which ranges from ten thousand to fifty thousand dollars. Overall, twenty thousand to sixty thousand dollars is an estimated cost for the complete service, including permanent storage and maintenance.

"There is not one itsy-bitsy piece of evidence to support the plaintiffs' claim regarding their deal with CSC. We have documentation signed by both Harrington brothers regarding their true donation to CSC. You will see that CSC did everything possible to continue Mrs. Harrington's suspension despite their lack of funds. This whole tragedy was an experiment, the capsule failure was an accident, and my client was no longer able to preserve her body.

"No one was at fault. There was absolutely no intent to cheat or defraud. All the money donated to CSC was used to bring about the desired results of both Mr. Nelson and Mrs. Harrington's sons. CSC is a nonprofit medical research foundation. I repeat, every suspension and all money received is a donation."

Winterbotham paused, his voice becoming softer and more reflective. "We live in an amazing age, full of medical miracles and possibilities. Everything attempted by Mr. Nelson was grounded in the possibilities proposed by top scientists, including the founder of cryonics, Professor Robert Ettinger, and using procedures developed by esteemed medical doctors. This was no snake oil salesman like the plaintiffs would wish you to believe. Nevertheless, cryonics is a long shot. There are no guarantees, and that is why donations are necessary to use these new procedures. The concept of relatives suing for every loved one not revived is truly insane."

My attorney went on to explain that we did not even have a permanent storage facility at that time, though we did expect to begin constructing one within two to three years.

"I certainly understand their love for their mother, but once Mrs. Harrington was in a capsule, all CSC could promise was their best efforts to keep her there. The Harringtons' responsibility included donating one hundred to three hundred dollars monthly to help with the liquid nitrogen charges. They never did that.

"CSC kept their promise: They froze her, they shipped her to California, and they kept her in dry ice for over two years. They got her into a capsule, and they maintained that capsule for over a year. CSC did what they said they would do." He stopped and pointed at the plaintiffs. "They did not."

That ended Winterbotham's presentation, which I thought had sufficiently neutralized Nothern's lies.

At that point the judge ordered a recess and invited the attorneys into his private chambers. After about forty-five minutes, they returned and resumed court. Winterbotham was red with anger and white-knuckled his briefcase. Something was very wrong, and I was suddenly frightened. *What the hell could have happened in there?* When I asked him in a nervous whisper, he mouthed, "Later," and swatted me away. I recoiled in shock, and he started laughing. After laughing and pointing at my stunned expression, he put his head in his hands, lowered his face to the table, and fell asleep!

As the jury was filing in and everyone else—spectators, clerks, deputies—was coming to attention, my slumbering attorney began snoring! It took a few minutes before everyone realized what was happening. I could hear Dennis Harrington sniggering, and I began to vigorously shake Winterbotham and yell at him to wake up. Klockgether's attorney, Mr. Freedman, whispered through clenched teeth, "Bob, get him up; this is making a terrible impression on the jury."

No shit.

I stole a quick look at the jury; they were stifling giggles. The judge banged his gavel and ordered the bailiffs to remove the jury. He then ordered them to wake up Winterbotham.

Good luck, I thought. *I couldn't do it.*

After fifteen minutes of cold water compresses to his face and being dragged to his feet, he finally began to respond. At first he was angry, almost combative, and was flailing his arms and yelling at everyone to leave him alone.

Thirty minutes elapsed before he could compose himself enough to properly explain what had just happened.

Judge Shelby took Winterbotham back into his chambers, alone this time. After thirty minutes my attorney came out looking pale and exhausted. He asked me to drive his car home.

For a long time on the freeway, I gripped the steering wheel, not speaking, awash with so many questions and concerns. Then I asked him one of the more benign questions: "What happened the first time you went into the judge's chambers with the other attorneys?"

He lifted his head and mumbled. His words were slurred, so I asked him to repeat them. This time he shouted, "The judge will not allow the AGA into evidence!"

My mind exploded with the ramifications, and I nearly veered our car into the other lane as I tried to absorb this death knell. The Anatomical Gift Act had been our security blanket for the past fifteen years. Without it, we never would have frozen anyone. We were now naked and exposed, without the legal protection we had operated under for years. I couldn't comprehend on what basis the AGA would not be allowed into evidence. It was a legal document, a contract, that the plaintiffs had agreed to and signed, and I had acted in good faith for all those years under the terms of the AGA. For me it made as much sense as a judge summarily and baselessly throwing out someone's marriage license or property deed.

"What," I finally said, flabbergasted, "are you nuts? That cannot be! That will kill our whole case." I had been thinking that the judge was leaning toward Nothern, and that had just confirmed it for me.

"I know," he said, rubbing his temples, I guessed to stay awake. "I'll have to figure out the basis for why he's barring the AGA, but it doesn't matter. I know I can beat this case without it. They have nothing but an unbelievable lie with no supporting evidence. Don't worry. I can do it. Besides, we'd win an appeal if we needed it."

A guarantee of a new trial offered little comfort—I could barely stomach this trial, let alone the prospect of a second one. I was in so much shock over the devastating bombshell, I never asked about his falling asleep. And unlike my lawyer, I'm sure, I couldn't sleep that night. I just paced my empty and lonely apartment for hours.

The next morning my lawyer looked refreshed and clear-eyed, and he smelled like clean linen and a pricey cologne I hadn't been able to buy for years. I didn't want to risk the positive mood of the day, so I didn't mention his bizarre behavior in court. I did comment on Nothern's skill, and he agreed, adding, "But we have the truth on our side."

He said he had spent half the previous evening checking the law books and consulting with other attorneys. He had checked our articles of incorporation, and, yes, we were authorized to carry out low-temperature research. The judge had decided incorrectly and had undercut our entire defense.

<hr/>

THE OFFENSE

We arrived at court when the jurors were settling in. Nothern struggled to his crutches and began, greeting the jury with a sincere smile. With that slow Southern lilt, he called his first witness, Mr. Troy Flower. He was an effeminate and seemingly nice young fellow, but I sat there paranoid and mostly confused about what he would say.

He testified that he had been a friend of the Harringtons for many years and was present when the brothers researched cryonics. They had contacted CSC, received information on the procedures, and were very excited about the hope it gave them to preserve their mother. They had purchased Professor Ettinger's book, *The Prospect of Immortality*, and my book, *We Froze the First Man*. He claimed he was present when the Harrington brothers made the business deal for their mother's suspension, and that it wasn't a donation.

"Mr. Nelson claimed he could bring Mrs. Harrington back to life just as soon as they could cure her cancer," Flower said. "He swore that ten thousand dollars was the total cost, and that's all there was to it." That was the end of Nothern's questioning.

It was now Winterbotham's turn to cross-examine Mr. Flower. He first asked, "How many times have you met Mr. Nelson?" Flower squirmed a bit, admitting he had never actually met me.

"Well, then," Winterbotham asked, "you never did actually hear Mr. Nelson speak to the Harrington brothers with your own two ears, did you?"

"Well, they told me exactly what Mr. Nelson promised and—"

"Hold on, Mr. Flower, this testimony is hearsay. You, of your own knowledge, know absolutely nothing about these discussions, do you, sir? And more important, your attorneys know that and had no business putting you on the stand other than to try and corrupt the integrity of these proceedings."

Flower looked blank, clueless as to how to answer.

"No further questions, sir."

Winterbotham later explained to me that Flower was just a ploy to set the stage for their first real witness, Terry Harrington. His entrance appeared as grand as a Broadway show. He flounced to the witness stand wearing a purple velvet cape that swung over the wooden divider and a silky, clinging shirt and purple pants. His hair was long and flowing. The jury loved it; they had been expecting a boring trial, not theater.

He had truly loved his mother, of that I was certain. Nothern took Terry step by step through the first moment he heard about cryonics to the reading of Ettinger and my books to the moment they placed the first call to CSC. Terry said he reached an answering service and left a message.

"Mr. Nelson called back in about twenty minutes. I explained that my mother was close to death; I guessed about two to four weeks. Mr. Nelson explained the procedures and the expense. He said ten thousand dollars would cover everything. He never mentioned a donation. If I wanted to proceed with my mother's suspension, we needed to make preparations and find a cooperating mortuary."

Hearing his testimony, I sighed. There was just enough truth mixed in with the lies and distortion to make his version seem plausible.

"He suggested he could come to Des Moines and complete the necessary arrangements. Mr. Nelson then came to Iowa and stayed about four days so that we could sign the paperwork and make all the preparations for my mother's freezing."

Nothern leaned on the jury box for support. He was angled so that when Terry spoke, the jury could see Terry's emotions play out on his expressive face. "You say you signed all the paperwork. Could you tell me exactly what you signed, and do you have any copies of what you signed?"

"I have no idea what I signed. I was so distraught I could not think clearly. And Mr. Nelson never gave me copies of what I signed. He promised he would send me copies, but he never did."

I scribbled a question on Winterbotham's yellow pad and poked it at his face, hoping he could decipher my shorthand.

"So you believed that once your mother arrived in California, your responsibility was over until the day your mother came walking back into your life even better than when she left?"

Terry pulled out a purple handkerchief and dabbed his eyes. "That is exactly correct, sir."

"Your witness, Mr. Winterbotham."

Winterbotham took a few minutes before he began his cross-examination. I think he wanted to raise the tension a little more. Finally he began. "Mr. Harrington, when Mr. Nelson arrived in Iowa, where did he stay?"

"At my home."

"So you had a leisurely amount of time to discuss matters and to talk. I mean, you were not under any kind of time restraint, is that correct?"

Terry nodded. "That's right."

"So in your discussions with Mr. Nelson, are you telling us that the question of donations never came up? You're telling this jury that this was just like any other purchase, maybe like buying a car or a boat, nothing unusual, just an ordinary business deal. Right?"

"It was not really anything unusual."

Winterbotham feigned exaggerated surprise for the jury's benefit. "Your mother is dying and you want to freeze her. By your own testimony, you were feeling so very distraught, and now you're saying it wasn't anything unusual?"

"Objection, counsel is badgering the witness."

Winterbotham spun toward Nothern. "I'd like to hear him answer the question."

"Sustained," said the judge, which ended the debate.

Winterbotham groaned and stuck out his lower lip. "Mr. Harrington, since you claim this was just an ordinary purchase of a service, would it be fair to refer to this transaction as a service agreement?"

Terry flounced his hair. "I think that would be fair."

"Then as you would receive in any ordinary purchase of a service agreement, would you show me a copy of that service agreement that you and your brother signed?"

"We never got a copy of that agreement. I already said that. Mr. Nelson promised to send me a copy of that agreement but never did."

I rolled my eyes at his response. Of course I had sent it.

"Would you then explain to me, Mr. Harrington, why I have here in my hand documents signed by you and your brother donating your mother's body and ten thousand dollars to the Cryonics Society of California?"

"I have no idea what I signed. I was so confused and distraught, I have no idea what those documents might have said. I am, however, positive that I would never donate my mother's body to anyone." Terry leaned forward and spoke louder. "Don't you understand? She's my mother!"

"I remind you, Mr. Harrington, you are under oath here today."

The plaintiffs' lawyer jumped up. "Objection!"

"Sustained," said the judge.

Winterbotham continued. "Up until the time of the accident at the CSC facility, would you agree that the service offered by CSC was adequate? Would you agree Mr. Nelson made every effort to comply with your wishes? Didn't the CSC make it possible for your family and friends from Iowa to see your mother in a memorial service after being frozen in dry ice for almost two years?"

"They did the best they could, I suppose."

"After the accident at Chatsworth, did Mr. Nelson come and see you at the airport in Des Moines?"

"Yes."

"Were you alone?"

"No, I was with my wife."

"Where did you meet Mr. Nelson?"

"We met at the gate and then went to a restaurant at the airport."

"Did Mr. Nelson tell you about the capsule failure at the CSC facility?"

"He may have mentioned it."

"Well, Mr. Harrington, I would think that you would remember something of this importance; either he did or he didn't mention it. I mean it wasn't as if he was just flying in by jumbo jet and decided to stop for a cup of coffee. It was obviously a very serious matter for him to go through the personal expense and effort to fly to Des Moines to talk to you face to face. I mean, if it wasn't very important, he could have just telephoned you, correct?"

"Well, yes, he did say there was a problem at the facility, something about the capsule failing for a few days. But I told him to just start it up again and keep on going. I have enormous faith in the future of science."

"Mr. Harrington, have you ever read any cryonics promotional material?"

"Yes. Mr. Nelson sent a packet to me prior to his arrival in Iowa."

"Did you read the material he sent you?"

"Yes, I looked at it briefly. I had already decided to freeze my mother, so I didn't feel the need to read every word."

"How about your brother? Wasn't he interested enough to read this unique material, to understand the arrangements surrounding this life-saving experiment for your mother? Are you sure, Mr. Harrington, that your self-serving loss of memory is not connected to your effort to extract a large financial settlement out of this lawsuit?"

"Objection! Your Honor, counsel is extremely argumentative," said Nothern.

"Sustained."

Winterbotham scowled. Worse still, the judge and jury saw it.

"So, Mr. Harrington, do I understand you correctly that even in the face of knowing all the other cryonics suspended patients in California are acknowledged medical donors, that all the frozen patients throughout the country are medical donors, and that no cryonics organization anywhere in the world will accept a patient for cryonic suspension unless through donation, you still claim you never heard about the medical donor requirement in order to be a candidate for becoming a cryonic suspension patient?"

"That's right; no one ever mentioned that."

I was thrilled and had to sit on my hands so that I wouldn't show my giddiness. *Go on, hang yourselves.* All the documentation was on our side.

"I have no more questions, Your Honor."

The next witness was Dennis Harrington. Dennis was muscular; he owned and taught at a karate school. He was a soft-spoken man who had also loved his mother.

Dennis stuck to the script and parroted everything his brother Terry had said. He added that he had wondered how CSC would be capable of bringing his mother back to life; it sounded very expensive. "Mr. Nelson said that with any luck, we should have her back in a few years."

Winterbotham raised his eyebrows and inched forward, poised for attack. "That's odd. Wasn't it stated earlier that Mr. Nelson promised to pay for the liquid nitrogen for a thousand years? So which is it—a few years or a thousand years?"

Dennis looked to his brother and, not receiving any help, merely shrugged.

"Mr. Harrington, why did you and your brother have your father removed from his grave in Iowa?"

"Mr. Nelson said it might even be possible to bring him back too."

"Yes, but your father had been dead for two years, autopsied, and embalmed."

"Mr. Nelson said there might be a few cells alive, and if we could find a couple we might be able to clone them."

I coughed to stifle a laugh. That assertion was so absurd, I couldn't comprehend how anyone could possibly believe it. I looked at the jury and saw them enraptured by his testimony. Sickening dread washed over me when I realized they believed him. This was not a good omen.

"Was your father frozen after he was delivered to the CSC storage vault?"

"No, he was not."

"Did they look for any *alive* cells?"

"No, they didn't."

"How much did it cost to transfer your father to your mother's cemetery?"

"It was three thousand dollars."

"And whom was the money paid to?"

"I don't know."

"Well, Mr. Harrington, I have a record here that shows that Terry and you paid three thousand dollars for mortuary services, which covered the removal from the ground in Iowa and the flight to California. There was no other purpose than to keep both of your parents at the same burial site."

Nothern stood up. "Is there a question forthcoming?"

Winterbotham turned and glared at him but continued. "Do you expect this jury to believe that Mr. Nelson actually suggested that science could revive your father *after he'd been autopsied?* And more important, Mr. Harrington, do you think anyone here today believes that even you could believe such nonsense could ever be possible?"

Dennis pointed a finger at me. "He made me believe it."

"Mr. Harrington, were you aware that Mr. Nelson gave a lecture to a group of doctors at the Iowa Memorial Hospital? The title of the talk was 'Death and the Dying Patient' and was arranged by your brother. He discussed how cryonics stalls the dying process after today's doctors have declared the patient legally dead. Then the CSC brings the patient far into the future for help not yet possible by today's medical science."

"I don't remember that talk exactly."

"You don't remember that cryonics was explained to those doctors exactly as Mr. Nelson explained it to you—as an all-volunteer, medical-donation enterprise whose idea was slowly spreading all across the country?"

"No, sir, I don't remember that."

"Did you know that Mr. Nelson has been on countless radio and television shows? He's explained that suspended animation is not guaranteed in any way to be successful. If someone is buried or cremated, only then can we be certain of their future."

Dennis responded with a blank stare.

"No more questions."

As Dennis exited the witness stand, I watched him intently, wondering how he could expect anyone to believe such lies.

All of a sudden I heard a *pssst*. I looked over to see Winterbotham's head down on the table. He was asleep again, snoring and now drooling! I was mortified. Joseph Klockgether shook Winterbotham's lapels, and I gave him sharp jabs with my elbows. The jury was laughing their collective ass off at him and, consequently, at me. The judge stared in disbelief and then banged the gavel for the bailiffs to remove the jury.

I couldn't believe my rotten luck. I could tell that Worthington was thinking the same thing—he couldn't believe *his* luck. Worthington, the Worm, grinned like a Cheshire cat and acted like he'd just won the lottery.

For five minutes the two bailiffs tried waking Winterbotham. Spectators were laughing, and the reporters were scribbling in their notepads. I sat there confounded, wondering what kept happening to my attorney. The judge looked pissed and *ordered* the bailiffs, "Wake him, clean him up, and drag him, if necessary, into my chambers."

The bailiffs were big men and looked strong, but Winterbotham was over six feet tall and more than two hundred pounds of dead weight. As the bailiffs lugged him to the restroom, his arms slung over their shoulders, he roused out of unconsciousness and struggled against their firm grip. He yelled and gnashed his teeth like a rabid dog. None of his grunts sounded intelligible though, and I just had to breathe fast.

The judge banged his gavel, attempting to restore some amount of order. Most of the gallery quieted, but he still had to speak over Winterbotham's growling. "When Mr. Winterbotham is able, will the attorneys come to my chambers? Mr. Nelson, will you come also?"

I was shocked, and so was Mr. Freedman, Klockgether's attorney. He told me in all his years practicing law, he had never heard of a defendant being asked to join the attorneys in chambers. "Bob, you should get rid of him. He is making a laughingstock out of you. Tell the judge you want to become your own attorney."

Thirty minutes later, Winterbotham returned to the courtroom. The bailiff opened the judge's door and ushered us in. After we were seated around an imposing oak table, the judge began. "Mr. Winterbotham, yesterday I gave you twenty-four hours to get your medication adjusted so that you could function in this trial, and you fell asleep right in the middle of a sentence."

"Yes, sir; I knew I'd need more for the trial, but I guess the doctor hasn't gotten the dosage right yet, Your Honor."

"Well, I'm going to give you one more chance to get it right, Mr. Winterbotham. If you don't, you're going to be found in contempt of court and will be sentenced to jail. This is your very last chance, do you understand me?"

My attorney nodded, drool stains still on his shirt. "Yes, sir, I do."

I jumped in and asked, "Wait a minute, what's going on here? What kind of medicine is he taking?"

The judge swung his head to me, and his eyes grew wide. He took a deep breath and said, "Are you telling me you don't know that Mr. Winterbotham is manic-depressive and takes lithium?" I could only shake my head. He turned to my attorney. "Mr. Winterbotham, you don't have a signed release from Mr. Nelson allowing you to represent him in your present condition?"

There was no response.

"Oh, boy," said the judge. After what seemed like an eternity, the judge looked at Nothern and said, "Let's get brutally honest here. What you and your clients are after is money, and unless I'm wrong, Mr. Nelson has none."

"That's right, Your Honor," I answered. "I had to sell my car just to pay Mr. Winterbotham to represent me."

The judge reminded the plaintiffs' attorneys that I had a guaranteed appeal because of Winterbotham's failure to obtain a written release to represent me while using lithium. I also had an equally good shot at a new trial because of the judge's denial to allow the Anatomical Gift Act to be introduced.

Well, this is an unexpected development, I thought. I was surprised at his candor and had assumed judges tried to avoid their decisions being overruled, since it might make them look bad. Obviously, with this judge, I was wrong.

"Now I would suggest that you gentlemen let Mr. Nelson out of this action and continue one against Mr. Klockgether, who has the malpractice insurance and the money you're after. Otherwise, even if you win against Mr. Nelson, you can't collect until after his appeal is heard and there is a new trial. Believe me, gentlemen, he will be granted a new trial."

Nothern and Worthington exchanged conflicted glances and asked the judge if they could have fifteen minutes in private. My one indulgence was enjoying the look of panic smear across Worthington's face as they left the room.

Those next fifteen minutes sitting in the judge's chambers felt like hundreds of years. It felt so long, I wouldn't have been surprised if reanimation had become possible during that interval. I couldn't look at Winterbotham or the judge. I just fidgeted, swallowed up by my deep leather chair. When the attorneys returned, they informed the judge they did not want to release me from the lawsuit. I learned later they felt they needed *me*, the General, to win their case. These guys were great chess players, and they had some brilliant moves planned.

I saw my opening and said, "Your Honor, I would like to make a motion here." I had never made a motion in my life. Before the judge could reply, I continued, "I would like to make a motion to fire my attorney and represent myself, on the grounds that he keeps falling asleep."

The judge looked at me with a barely concealed grin. "I'm sorry, Mr. Nelson. I cannot allow that, but if he falls asleep one more time . . . well, we will see what happens then. That's all for today."

The ride home was a nightmare from hell. Winterbotham looked like a pale, unblinking zombie from a horror movie, and I felt like one of his captured victims. I think he was so addlepated that it didn't register with him that I had asked the judge for permission to fire him. We didn't speak a word, and when we arrived at his house, I jumped out of the car without a good-bye and jogged to my vehicle.

That night I tried to sleep, but my eyes remained wide open as I wondered how much crazier this trial could get. I had never before been in a sinking vortex where things kept spinning faster and faster out of control. I could not comprehend that my attorney, who had gotten my last nickel, was mentally ill and taking lithium, which causes people to fall sleep. People on this medication should not be representing clients in court.

This manic-depressive was representing me, fighting for my honor, my reputation, and my financial future. Yes, he was fighting for my fucking life.

And he was nuts.

On the other side of the courtroom aisle, there was Mr. Nothern, who was so smooth and beguiling that he could convince my mother to side with the plaintiffs. And even more unbelievable, I liked him.

The next morning I had simmered down. I resigned myself to just riding this nutso trial to its conclusion and then deciding how to proceed with my life. Winterbotham always looked great in the morning but deteriorated as the court session went on. He thought I would take the stand that day. We arrived at 8:45 a.m., and court began at 9:00 a.m.

The next witness for the plaintiffs was Marie Brown, Louis Nisco's daughter, who wanted her own piece of the malpractice pie. Years earlier she had called CSC and begged me to move her father's capsule to our Chatsworth facility so that Ed Hope wouldn't kick his body into the street. She essentially testified that I had agreed to pick up her father's capsule and replace the liquid nitrogen for free, forever! That was all Marie offered the court.

Her statements were another pinprick to my soul, an additional betrayal of my decade of service and sacrifice.

Winterbotham asked why anyone would go through all the work and enormous expense of picking up that capsule, moving it to California, storing it, and replacing liquid nitrogen for perhaps centuries. "All of that free of charge," he said. "Did that make any sense to you, Ms. Brown?"

She shrugged. "I just thought they wanted to do that."

"You just thought they wanted to accept this responsibility forever for free; that is your testimony before this court today?"

"Yes, sir."

"How much money did you give Mr. Nelson?"

No answer.

"It was zero. How much did *he* pay on your behalf?"

"Fifteen hundred dollars," she replied after an interminable pause.

"He was doing you a favor. He rescued your father." He pointed his finger at her. "You washed your hands of your father's care, and Mr. Nelson stepped up. Isn't that what really happened?"

No answer.

"Please answer the question."

She said softly, "He deceived me."

I tried handing Winterbotham her handwritten note that she had sent me after I took charge of her father's capsule. I glanced through the flowery cursive she had sent me then as I listened to her testimony; the startling disconnect wounded me yet again.

Mr. Nelson,

This letter is about my father's care and continued suspension. I am simply unable to find the money to help keep his suspension going. At this point in time, I am donating the capsule and my father to the Cryonics Society of California, and whatever happens will be in your hands. I am unable to donate any money whatsoever. At this point in time, I find it necessary to walk away from this responsibility. I wish you good luck and thank you with all my heart for your amazing work in the field of cryonic suspension.

Best wishes,
Marie Brown

I willed Winterbotham to keep pushing her for the truth, but he didn't. He spun on his heel, stomped back to our table, and sat down.

With that, the plaintiffs rested their case.

◦ ◦ ◦

THE DEFENSE

Winterbotham called me as his first witness for the defense. As I stood with my hand on the Bible being sworn in, I looked across the courtroom and noticed he was laughing. A few minutes earlier he had been glowering, as though he might kill someone.

He sat at the conference table, swinging his legs and giggling like a schoolkid. The judge waited for several minutes before asking if he was ready to proceed with questioning me. Winterbotham snapped to and stood up, but he was still laughing, presumably at me. *Oh, God*, I thought. *What am I doing here? Am I the laughingstock of this entire courtroom?*

I was upset. I had hoped my testimony could salvage my case and convince the jury I hadn't deceived anyone. Instead, the focus was entirely on my attorney and his mood swings.

His first question was: "Mr. Nelson, what do you do for a living?"

"I'm an electronics technician, and I own my own business, which gave me the opportunity to function at CSC as president."

"Mr. Nelson, are you a scientist, an inventor, or a doctor?"

"No, I am not, sir."

"Then how were you qualified to run a cryonics society and freeze people?" His question had a harsh, sarcastic edge.

I could not believe what the son-of-a-bitch was doing to me! He was treating me like a hostile witness! Well, I had to go on—hoping it would get better.

I said, "It's a matter of faith, Mr. Winterbotham. If you believe—no, strike that—if I believe in something, I give it 100 percent of my support. I felt like this was my calling. Does that make any sense?"

"Certainly it does." Winterbotham looked at the jury. "Certainly it does. Would you explain to this jury how you became involved in cryonics?"

I answered that I attended one of the first meetings about low-temperature biology as it applies to human beings. After CSC was formed and I was elected president, I enlisted professionals to help discover reliable methods of human suspended animation.

"Tell us, Mr. Nelson, how much money did you or CSC receive for freezing the first man, Dr. James Bedford?"

"We never received a single penny or a thank-you. As a matter of fact, CSC paid for all the chemicals, the dry ice, and a specially constructed storage container. We also paid for transportation, ten days' storage, and the delivery of Dr. Bedford's body to his son, Norman."

"Who was the next person frozen by CSC?"

"That was Marie Sweet. She was a valued and active member of CSC."

"When did Marie Sweet get suspended?"

"August 27, 1967."

"How much money did CSC receive for Ms. Sweet's suspension?"

"We received three hundred dollars; that was all the money the family had to their name. She and her husband, Russ Van Norden, lived on Social Security. Professor Ettinger also donated one hundred dollars for Marie."

"Tell us, Mr. Nelson, about the next cryonics freezing."

"That was Ms. Helen Kline. Helen was the first person I ever spoke to about human suspended animation."

"When was Ms. Kline suspended?"

"On May 14, 1968."

"How much money did the CSC receive for Ms. Kline's suspension?"

"We received one hundred dollars one month before she passed away. I knew Ms. Kline was penniless."

"Well, Mr. Nelson, it doesn't appear that this scam, as Mr. Nothern calls it, is producing any big money! I mean, the first three suspensions brought in a grand total of five hundred dollars."

Winterbotham looked at the jury as though he didn't understand, hoping they would question the seeming contradiction.

"Tell us about the next freezing."

"That was Mr. Russell Stanley. Russ was the Cryonics Society historian. He had collected every written word about cryonics from across the country and talked to every person who even thought about cryonics."

"When was Mr. Stanley suspended?"

"That was on September 6, 1968."

"And how much money did the Society receive for Mr. Stanley's suspension?"

"CSC received a ten-thousand-dollar donation from the Stanley estate."

"What did CSC do with that money?"

"Over the next three years, we paid out in excess of ten thousand dollars for replacement of dry ice for the temporary storage of Marie Sweet, Helen Kline, and Russ Stanley."

"Tell us about the next suspension."

"That was Ms. Mildred Harrington."

"Was there anything unusual about the Harrington suspension?"

"Nothing other than that she lived in Des Moines, Iowa, and her sons didn't have enough money for perpetual care. CSC agreed to do the complete suspension, including placement in a capsule, at which time the brothers agreed to make a monthly donation of one hundred to three hundred dollars. This was not mandatory, but the commitment was part of our agreement."

"What did CSC do with the money it received from the Harringtons? Was it a donation or a private business deal between you and Terry Harrington on the side?"

"No, it was just like every other suspension. I couldn't proceed otherwise. We had many expenses with Mrs. Harrington—creating the dry ice container, furnishing it with dry ice, making the vault safe to store a dry ice box down in it, placing Mrs. Harrington in a capsule when we were fortunate enough to receive it, replenishing the liquid nitrogen."

"Will you examine these documents, Mr. Nelson, and tell me if these are the papers you and the Harrington brothers signed, donating the body of Mrs. Harrington and the ten thousand dollars to CSC?"

"Yes, those are the exact documents we signed in Des Moines."

I watched the faces of each juror. *Don't they understand?* This was a basic contract. We had the same protection afforded to medical students dissecting people in their gross anatomy class.

"Who was the next cryonics patient, Mr. Nelson?"

"Genevieve de la Poterie. She was a seven-year-old child from Canada. She was dying from a Wilms tumor on her kidney. Her parents had no money, and I just fell in love with this sweet little girl. At that time I had a daughter just two years older than this beautiful angel."

"How much did CSC receive from that suspension?"

"Not a penny. In fact, I donated one thousand dollars of my own money for her suspension."

Winterbotham paused, hoping that testimony would be remembered in the jury room.

"Well, Mr. Nelson, something is missing here. Where is the scam part, the part where you con everyone out of their fortunes? So far it looks like you're the one being conned. You're the one receiving tons of work, responsibility, and debt along with horrible accusations that you're stealing unbelievable sums of these people's money."

As Winterbotham said that, he slammed his book down on the defense table. Then he screamed, "Where is the money, Mr. Nelson? Where are you hiding it?"

Judge Shelby pounded his gavel, several people in the gallery woke up, and I didn't know whether to laugh or cry. It was bizarre, but I think he made his point. A little nutty maybe, but well done!

"So, Mr. Nelson, you've got all these people frozen in different locations. Who's paying for all these expenses—pumps, liquid nitrogen, dry ice, traveling every day to the vault and then to Buena Park and the temporary storage facility? Capsules breaking down, meetings, fly here, fly there. Who is paying for all this activity, Mr. Nelson? Who's paying all these bills?"

All his questions made me defensive and I stammered, "I did the best I could for as long as possible."

"Mr. Nelson, tell us about the day you returned to the Chatsworth vault to find the pump not running and the capsules hot, sitting in a hundred-degree-plus sun. Who was in the capsule at that time?"

"Mildred Harrington, Steven Mandell, and Genevieve de la Poterie. I was quite worried about the capsule and its patients. I had made arrangements with the cemetery's groundskeeper to call the Gilmore cryogenic company if there was any problem." I stopped for a minute; it was tough recounting that horrible day.

"When I drove up to the capsule, I could see that the pump was off with no vapor discharging from the valve. It took me a long time to muster the courage to touch the exhaust. Finally I got up enough nerve to check; the pipe was hot, and I mean burning hot. I gasped and fell to my knees and cried. I had failed them, all of them." I stopped to take a breath. "I failed them."

"Your witness," Winterbotham said.

It was now Nothern's turn to twist the knife. I actually looked forward to it. After all, if I was the horrible person that he claimed, it should be simple for this sharp attorney to chew me up. I was ready for him.

"Mr. Nelson, how are you today, sir?"

"I've had better days."

"Well, sir, you're holding up very well. This must be a great strain for you."

He caught me off guard with his concern. He was playacting for the jury or had something quite sinister waiting for me.

"Mr. Nelson, I understand that after Mrs. Harrington had been frozen for over a year, you and Mr. Klockgether allowed Terry and Dennis Harrington to have a viewing for the family and friends of their mother."

"I believe ten or so guests came to California for that event, and, might I add, they were profoundly comforted by it."

"Was that to your knowledge, Mr. Nelson, the first time in history that a person who had been deceased for over a year had been viewed publicly?"

"With the exception of the Russian leader Lenin and Disney's Sleeping Beauty," I checked the jury to make sure they got my joke, "I believe it was."

"And, Mr. Nelson, if I understand you correctly, you claim the Harrington brothers had promised to make monthly donations to help with their mother's liquid nitrogen costs, is that true?"

"Yes, that is true."

Nothern leaned over the witness box. I could see the glint in his eye and half-hidden smile. Despite his impeccable manners, he enjoyed the hunt as much as Worthington. "I believe the preparations for the memorial were quite elaborate. It involved fabricating a new cryogenic system that sprayed liquid nitrogen to keep the body cooled enough for two hours."

"Yes; Mr. Klockgether worked hard to make the service as perfect as possible."

"How did Mrs. Harrington look, Mr. Nelson?"

"Her sons had taken a great deal of effort to prepare her; they spent hours getting her ready. Several times I had to shut the casket to allow it to cool down again."

Nothern got a twinkle in his eye, and I braced myself for his punch line.

"Well, Mr. Nelson, if you claim the Harrington brothers promised to make donations each month and never made even one, why would you go through all this trouble and expense on their behalf? And why would you not even mention this failed promise?"

I easily countered his coup de grâce. "It was not a problem since, at that time, she was in temporary storage. The donations were not scheduled to begin until Mrs. Harrington was placed into a capsule. Also, we charged the Harringtons an additional five thousand dollars for the memorial services, which they paid in advance. It was an exceptional event, and they got more than their money's worth."

Nothern had tried to sandbag me, but even with my easy deflection, he managed to look unscathed. He asked me next if I thought there could have been some simple misunderstanding about Mrs. Harrington being donated to CSC. "I mean, you were asking them to not only give away ten thousand dollars, but you asked for their mother as well."

I glanced over to Winterbotham for his silent direction, but he wasn't listening. Instead he was drinking glass after glass of water.

"We made the same presentation to everyone across the country who wanted our help for a cryonic suspension. It is the only legal structure that will provide some degree of protection against these types of lawsuits."

"Thank you; that is all."

Winterbotham then called his next witness, Marcelon Johnson, who had been the treasurer of CSC and had become my good fairy when she took over as president when I had to resign. Winterbotham asked about her duties as the CSC treasurer. She explained she kept track of membership dues and planned speaking engagements.

"We were an all-volunteer society. We knew our president, Bob Nelson, was honest, hardworking, and a true believer in the science of cryonics." She stopped and flashed me a gorgeous smile. "The cryonics time machine can bring us to a future generation who can save our precious gift of life."

Nothern on cross-examination asked only two questions of Ms. Johnson: first, whether she was aware if I ever used my own money to pay for cryonics expenses. She said, "Yes, we have all done that."

The next question concerned what she knew about the financing of the long-term storage vault at Chatsworth and how many people remained in that vault.

She answered, "I have no idea. That was something Mr. Nelson handled exclusively. He did not want others involved because of its highly experimental nature."

With that, Nothern had no further questions.

The next witness was the great Marshall Neel. Marshall was deeply involved in every aspect of the cryonics movement, and I still saw him often.

"Mr. Neel, what was your involvement in the Cryonics Society of California?"

"I was a business advisor for the program. I am now a teacher and public relations director for the Long Beach Water Company. I have long lent my expertise to benevolent organizations that I support in my private life."

"Is cryonics an organization you support with your whole heart?"

"Yes, I can say yes to that."

"What do you think of Mr. Nelson's contribution to CSC over these past years?"

"I think Mr. Nelson gave CSC all he's got and more. That dedication and drive is what landed him in this courtroom today. There comes a time when you have to let go of a burden if you want to survive." Marshall's words rolled out like silk. "Mr. Nelson would not let go."

"How much money were you paid by CSC?"

"Nothing. Nor was any other member."

"Do you intend to be frozen yourself, Mr. Neel?"

"That, sir, is my personal business, and I respectfully decline to answer that question."

"What was your contribution to CSC?"

"I was simply available whenever an opinion on a particular action was needed. I often gave talks for membership promotion."

"What was your official position?" Winterbotham asked, and then he started laughing. Marshall looked surprised, while Joseph and I exchanged questioning glances. My esteemed attorney kept tittering as he walked back to the defense table and sat down. No one wanted to laugh with him, and the awkward moment stretched out interminably as the moments clicked by. Finally I elbowed him in his gut.

"Right," Winterbotham said as he hopped out of his chair with so much energy, his feet came off the floor. He took a big gulp of water from his glass and bounded back to the witness.

"Mr. Neel, tell me about Cryonic Interment, the for-profit corporation started, I believe, by you and Mr. Nelson? What was its purpose?"

Marshall sat tall in the witness chair. "CI was a legal structure to assist CSC in purchasing equipment and offering cryonic services."

"Whatever became of Cryonic Interment?"

"Nothing. CSC never got far in obtaining patients who could afford to have their bodies cryonically suspended. All but two of CSC's patients could not afford the procedure."

"So did CI conduct any business at all?"

"No, there was never a single transaction whatsoever by CI. There's not much use having a for-profit corporation when there aren't any *profits*."

"What role did you play in CSC's decision whether to freeze a patient?"

"I never offered advice. This was Mr. Nelson's decision alone. No one else wanted any responsibility for the frozen remains of people who did not arrange adequate financing for their suspension."

"Were you in any way consulted about the Mildred Harrington cryonic suspension?"

"No, I was never asked about any cryonic suspension."

"No more questions."

Winterbotham's next witness was the great lady herself, Stella Gramer. She glided to the stand, statuesque and proud, with a crown of beautiful red hair and dressed in one of her many impeccably tailored suits. Although Stella was in her mid-eighties, she had a regal finesse and mental prowess that proved ageless.

I was honored to call her a great friend. Worthington had spent months trying to draw her into this lawsuit. He had subpoenaed her, deposed her, had private investigators spy on her, and attempted every possible dirty trick but never came close to entangling her in his shameful lawsuit.

Winterbotham introduced her by summarizing her illustrious career. She had been the youngest female attorney to pass the bar in California and had won the first huge judgment against the railroad for using illegal workers. She was a multimillionaire who had lived next door to Marilyn Monroe and was saddened by the apparent suicide of such a sweet woman.

He asked about our relationship. She said we had met at Holmby Park in Beverly Hills some twenty years before. She was watching her two young grandchildren play on the monkey bars, and I was walking my German shepherd puppy. The grandchildren and the puppy bonded instantly, as did we.

Winterbotham asked Stella about the cryonics program. She replied, "Beyond having an interest in the science, I didn't have a role. Mr. Nelson was kind enough to present me with *The Prospect of Immortality* by Professor Robert Ettinger. It was a wonderful book; I could see the absolute logic in it and for some time even considered it for myself."

"Have you then changed your mind about cryonic suspension?"

"I would say not for others, but I fear I am too set in my thinking to change. When I see the results of people fighting to get money and saying anything to get it, I would rather not subject my grandchildren to such a traumatic ordeal. They are what I live for today, and I think cryonics will be the wave of the future."

"Were you the official attorney for the CSC?"

"No. I mean, I never got paid or anything like that. Mr. Nelson is a very dear friend, and occasionally he asked me for an opinion or help in filling out a complicated legal form. Whatever I could do to help Mr. Nelson was my pleasure. But I never served in any official capacity."

I smiled at her as she perched on the edge of the witness stand. Hearing her take my part was one of the few bright spots in the trial; this ordeal certainly showed me who my real friends were.

"Did you help the Cryonics Society obtain its nonprofit status in California?"

"Yes, I did."

"I have no more questions, Ms. Gramer. I thank you for appearing here today on behalf of my client, and it's truly a pleasure to meet you."

Winterbotham was acting well, and I got to hear nice compliments from my friends. This was feeling like a good day—so far.

Now it was Nothern's turn, but sadly for me, he was too smart to try tackling her. She could easily parry any attack, and the plaintiffs did not want to risk their case by allowing her to make the defense look better. Nothern did, however, have a few questions.

He asked first if she had been the mysterious provider of the beautiful office suite in Westwood that was donated to CSC for three years. She responded, "Yes, I suppose I was."

Nothern shook his head. "Ms. Gramer, I can't for the life of me understand how you got yourself mixed up with such a crazy scam as freezing dead bodies."

She looked like she needed to educate him. "Well, Mr. Nothern, it is quite obvious that you have not read Professor Ettinger's book. I suggest you do. I think you'll have a very different opinion of cryonics once you have properly prepared for this case."

As she exited the witness stand, I wanted to blow her a kiss. I was feeling confident as the judge adjourned for lunch. There was a bottleneck of people at the exit, so I stopped off at the water fountain until the crowd cleared.

Two women, well dressed and in their thirties, sat on a nearby bench. Since getting divorced, I had started dating again, but I was a little too shy to approach them. I still felt inexperienced, since Elaine had been my first girlfriend and we had married as teenagers. Besides, a trial for my life was not an appropriate time to start flirting. They looked intelligent, though, and might see the logic of cryonics. I edged closer, trying to catch their eyes with a smile so that I could introduce myself.

I overheard the short-haired blond say to her friend, "I knew this cryonics stuff was nothing but a scam. Those poor families. He was just setting himself up as a new Messiah."

Her friend leaned in and countered, "It's worse than that. I heard he murdered people just so he could freeze them. He belongs in jail."

Messiah? Murderer? Jail? I bit my lip, stunned, and drew back. I could see someone believing I was negligent or a zealot, but how could anyone possibly accept such lies? *Did the jury think that too?* I started breathing fast as I glimpsed how effectively Worthington had sunk his fangs into my legacy. He was willing to destroy me by distorting this case far beyond a simple contract dispute. These women were strangers, completely unrelated to the trial, and yet they were convinced I was a criminal.

The women heard my loud exhale and turned toward me. I was seething. The blond's eyes grew wide; she quickly motioned to her friend and they skedaddled toward the cops in the lobby.

I collapsed on one of the hallway benches, completely dejected, and I sat there unmoving for the entire lunch break. My friend of twenty years, Sandra Stanley, was slated as the next witness and noticed me as she walked through the crowd. I couldn't explain, and I didn't need to; she wrapped her arms around my shoulders, gave me a quick hug, and led me into the courtroom.

Awhile back, Sandra had told me that when she was forty she wanted to study law. I told her she was nuts and that she would never make it. "Pick another profession," I had advised. Weeks earlier, Sandra had passed the bar exam on her first attempt, with the third-highest score of any applicant that year. Thankfully she never held my abysmal advice against me. Sandra had been a very strong supporter of cryonics since its inception. She was a fantastic writer and responded to thousands of inquiries to the CSC, published the cryonics newsletter, and cowrote my first book, *We Froze the First Man.*

Winterbotham guided Sandra through all the years she volunteered for the Cryonics Society. He then asked her to explain what the organization meant for her.

She replied, "We were participating in an epochal moment in which Professor Robert Ettinger had proclaimed to the world that the era of human death on Earth was about to come to an end."

He then asked her to comment on my character. She placed a hand over her heart and said, "Bob Nelson is one of the most sincere human beings I have ever had the pleasure to know in my life."

I gave her a half-smile, trying to forget the women in the hallway and instead focus on her words. She knew me and knew the truth.

"Thank you, Ms. Stanley. No more questions."

Nothern began his cross-examination. "Ms. Stanley, as a *very* close friend to Mr. Nelson and a trusted member of the CSC, did you know what was going on at the storage vault in Chatsworth?"

Sandra glowered and wagged her finger at Nothern. I had to grin— I'd wanted to do that a dozen times. "I don't know what you mean by 'going on.' That cemetery vault is where the cryonics patients were interred."

"What I am asking you, Ms. Stanley, is did you know exactly which persons were frozen and which ones were not and why?"

"At different times, I believe I did, but that constantly changed as equipment failed and patients were moved. Mr. Nelson did not want others involved in that quagmire." Sandra was speaking fast; she had an agenda for her testimony and a lot she wanted to say. "His life's goal was to save those patients; he considered them historically vital pioneers of the cryonics movement. If he had known he would be blamed if he failed, I think he would have done it anyway."

"Well, Ms. Stanley, how do you explain the loss of the Harrington brothers' mother and the ten thousand dollars they gave to Mr. Nelson?"

"The money was paid to the Cryonics Society of California as a donation supporting low-temperature biology and not to Mr. Nelson personally. It was certainly not a business deal, as you are trying to suggest."

"So what do you suggest, Ms. Stanley? Should we just accept this loss and let Mr. Nelson perpetuate this same scam on countless people across the country?"

"Mr. Nelson never scammed anybody." A strand of her long brown hair fell in her face, and she reached up to push it back. I could tell from her twitching hand that she needed a cigarette. "And he has resigned from CSC. Yes, there will undoubtedly be more losses in the future. However, you don't stop great scientific effort because someone didn't make it. Look at the first heart transplants. Look at the space program: They had losses, but no one gave up because of those failures. They took their losses, learned their lessons, and kept trying until they succeeded."

Nothern moved to align with the jury box. "It is clear, Ms. Stanley, that you have little compassion for these two young men's suffering and their enormous loss. You are a true believer in this body-freezing craze, which has absolutely no support from the medical or scientific communities whatsoever."

I elbowed Winterbotham and he sprang to his feet. "Objection . . . I mean, counsel should be asking questions, not making speeches."

Before the judge could sustain, Nothern said, "I have no more questions."

Sandra shook her finger at him again. "Mr. Nothern, scientists began the cryonics movement, and they are leading us into a brave, new world—"

"I said no more questions. You're excused."

Sandra blew her hair from her face, obviously frustrated and disappointed.

I looked at my attorney, hoping he would ask Sandra more questions on redirect examination. It didn't help our case having Nothern's statements ringing in the jury's ears. As Sandra rose to exit the witness stand, I knew that was a lost cause. Winterbotham had resumed his habit of resting his chin in his palm and staring off at Lady Justice.

Our next witness was Joseph Mendoza. Joe was the groundskeeper at the Chatsworth cemetery and had helped me with the vault. As he was sworn in, Joe was nervous and couldn't keep his voice from shaking and his hands from trembling; I felt bad that I needed him to testify.

Winterbotham began by yelling at him. I groaned. Of all our witnesses, Joe needed kid-glove handling. Yet Winterbotham continued, almost screaming. "What was your responsibility to the Cryonics Society?"

It seemed Winterbotham thought that by shouting at him, Joe would understand him better. The problem was that Joe knew my name but was unfamiliar with the term "Cryonics Society." He looked green, so I signaled Winterbotham back to our table; the judge ordered a half-hour recess.

I was thankful for that break. "Mr. Winterbotham," I whispered, "Joe is our witness; you shouldn't be shouting at him. The man is already scared to death just being here." I spent most of the recess trying to counsel my attorney about the best way to handle Joe. When court resumed, the questioning went much smoother. He asked Joe how long he had known me and if I was a good guy. These questions settled Joe a bit before he launched into describing the painful capsule failure to the jury.

When Joe finished his recounting of that sad day, he said, "I'm sorry for Mr. Bob; he's a very nice man."

"Mr. Mendoza, did you see Mr. Nelson at the cemetery very often?"

"I see Mr. Bob every day; sometime he come he stay all day. He work very hard to take care of everything."

"Your witness, Mr. Nothern."

Joe stiffened his shoulders, preparing himself for cross-examination.

"Mr. Mendoza, did Mr. Nelson tell you what was inside those capsules?"

"Well, he not tell me exactly, but I know what inside. We all know it's frozen people."

"Did you realize when you did nothing after the pump stopped that the people inside were lost forever?"

"I don't know; those people are dead. They can't die again."

"Was Mr. Nelson attentive to the capsules and the storage vault?"

"He came every day, bringing the smoking ice. He pump the water out of the vault; he blow the fan inside down there. He work very hard every day."

"Did you see other people trying to find out what is going on inside that vault?"

"People from the TV station came with a big camera. They break the lock and open the vault. We call police. I didn't like them for that."

"I have no more questions, sir."

Our final witness was a character to behold. Frank Farrell had been indispensable to me for years and a genius at resolving the never-ending problems at the vault.

Ever since we met, Frank absolutely would not conform to any kind of dress code. Regardless of the occasion, he wore outfits like green pants with a purple-and-pink shirt. Once I noticed he had on one red sock and one yellow sock.

Just for fun, I commented on it. He replied, "I know. I have another pair exactly like them at home."

I had pleaded with him to wear a suit to court. I explained that his entire credibility would depend on his appearance. As Frank walked to the witness stand, my face broke from apprehension into a big grin. I beamed with pride to see him dressed properly. His blue tie matched his blue suit, but it was tied so that it hung backwards. The whole ensemble looked as though he had just taken it out of the washing machine and wrung it out by hand, but it was a suit.

Winterbotham first asked Frank to tell the jury about his background and experience in the business world. Despite his appearance, Frank was quite a qualified engineer with an impressive education.

Winterbotham asked him about his connection to me. "I'm a fan of Bob Nelson and his effort to revive the people who were in cryonic suspension. He brought that vault into existence, and I know someday he'll be recognized for his great contribution to the world."

"Did Mr. Nelson pay you for your work?"

"Yes, he did."

Winterbotham transformed; he yelled at Frank. "How did he pay you, with CSC money or his own check?"

Frank's eyes got wide, but he maintained his calm. "Nope; I don't accept checks because I don't have a bank account. He always paid me in good ol' cash on the barrel."

Winterbotham shouted again. "Were you ever in that vault?"

"Hell, yes, about a thousand times or better. Whenever it was time to replace the dry ice on different patients, I was the one that helped him. I pumped water out of the facility at least once a week, and I helped him move bodies."

"What was your role?"

Frank paused because he'd just answered that, and Winterbotham shouted even louder than before. "I'm asking you a question! Don't you understand? *What did you do?*"

Frank drew back, surprised at the ferocity. This was just too crazy. I stood up and motioned Winterbotham back to the table. "What are you doing?" I whispered to him. "He's our witness."

That seemed to work. Winterbotham switched back to normal and spoke calmly to Frank. "So you've actually seen these frozen human beings?"

"I sure have, and Mr. Nelson took care of them as if they were his own family."

"May I ask you, Mr. Farrell, what does a frozen person look like after years of being frozen?"

"Compared to what? I mean, they certainly don't look alive, but they look like they could be revived if we only knew how to revive them. I guess that's what the CSC is all about. I don't know anyone else in the world who could've done the job that Mr. Nelson has done, and done it with hardly any money. I have a great respect for him and his effort. That's why I have always been there for him, and that's why I'm here for him today."

"Is there anything you can think of that Mr. Nelson could have done to prevent this tragedy at the cemetery?"

Frank fidgeted and tugged at his tie, uncomfortable in his court duds. "Sure, in hindsight I could think of a lot of things; you could do that about almost anything. Bob was running this operation by the seat of his pants. Always hoping someone would come along and provide some help in the form of money. Hell, he had a beautiful thirty-man capsule sitting up on that hill in Chatsworth manufactured by real cryogenic fabricators. That unit cost one hundred thousand dollars retail and sat on those grounds for three years. All he needed was the money to purchase a bigger vault and then get that capsule up and running. CSC would have been solvent for many years if they had not frozen a dozen people for free. We worked our butts off and gave it everything we had. We did a job we can be proud of."

"I thank you, Mr. Farrell. I have no more questions."

As Nothern made his way to the witness box on his crutches, he asked, "While Mr. Nelson was back East for two weeks, why did he not leave you in charge of checking those capsules every day, as he had typically done?"

"I guess you'd have to ask him that, but I venture to guess that since I live in Santa Monica and have no automobile, it would be a real chore and expense for me to go back and forth to the cemetery every day. It was about fifty miles and a drive through Topanga Canyon. Mr. Nelson always picked me up, and that was one hell of a trek. I wouldn't want to do it solo."

"Were you, Mr. Farrell, aware that the first capsule placed in the vault had failed and was no longer being filled with liquid nitrogen?"

"I was."

"What did Mr. Nelson say about that?"

"As I understood it, Mr. Nelson had been filling that capsule for a year or two. The capsule became less and less efficient, until it was just impossible to find the money to continue filling it. These Cryo-Care units were just not holding up like they needed to. It was a learning curve. We were just hanging in there until we could get that big beauty of a capsule up and running. Had that happened, none of us would be here today."

"Did you know when the second capsule containing the seven-year-old child and my clients' mother failed?"

"Yep, but I never heard from Bob after that loss. I think he just reached his breaking point and gave up. Then you guys came running after him for money. I guess that was the last straw."

"Thank you, Mr. Farrell."

That was the end of testimony.

In Summation

Nothern gave his closing argument first. He made even more of a performance than usual of getting himself up on his crutches and moving over to the front of the jury box.

Before he began, he first made eye contact with each jury member. "Good morning, ladies and gentlemen; it's a pleasure to see your bright and smiling faces this morning. I'm sure each of you is pleased to see the end of this case so that you can return to your family and your regular daily activities. I promise I will not keep you very long, and I sincerely thank you for being such an attentive group. Well, my friends, what we have here is a TV repairman posing as a great scientist. He was able to scam Terry and Dennis Harrington out of their entire inheritance left to them by their beloved mother.

"There is nothing else you can call what Mr. Nelson did to these two brothers that had just lost their mother, their most precious treasure, to cancer. Mr. Nelson descends on bereft, grief-stricken families and promises to take away their pain and loss."

He paused—wanting that little tidbit to sink in. I saw a few jurors exchange glances and raise their eyebrows. "This miracle group's leader set himself up as the General and claimed he could save the Harrington brothers' mother from death. Yes, the General had the power to bring back the dead! Now the only other person I know who could bring people back from the dead was Jesus Christ, and he doesn't look anything like Jesus Christ to me. Does he to you?"

Nothern raised his voice, and from his tone, he reminded me of one of those TV preachers. He pointed his forefinger at me, accusing me, smiting me. I could feel the stares from the jury. "As a matter of fact, he was better than Jesus Christ. He could bring everyone back from the dead—all he needed was your money."

Nothern stopped to let that little gem, the cornerstone statement of his entire case, sink into the jury's psyches. My blood went cold. I finally glimpsed their strategy—how every question, every fabrication, had built up to this deduction.

"Mr. Nelson not only promised he could bring Mrs. Harrington back from death, he said he could make her young again. Yes, can you imagine that he was going to make Mrs. Harrington twenty-one again?

"So they gave the General their last penny, all their trust, and their precious mother to care for until, the General promised, he would bring her back alive as a twenty-one-year-old beauty. He promised he could do all that for ten thousand dollars. The problem is, my friends, this is the biggest bunch of nonsense I ever heard in my life."

No, I thought, this *is the biggest bunch of nonsense ever.*

"I mean it. I could never even imagine that anyone would stoop so low as to fabricate such a preposterous pile of crap and then dupe grief-stricken survivors into buying it. The General was starting a new kind of religion, with himself as the leader and with the power to decree who shall live and who shall die. Just let your money do the talking. What do you think, ladies and gentlemen, do you think the General was, as Sandra Stanley put it, sincere?" Nothern slowly shook his head, answering his own question.

"So, my friends, what do we do here today? Do we give the General a pat on the back and say, 'Good job, General; go get some more poor fools' money'? Do we encourage this kind of treatment of our fellow Americans across the country? Because that's where these folks will take this insanity; they have even started cryonics societies in England, France, and several Latin American countries."

I heard a clatter of whispering behind me, but Judge Shelby didn't raise his gavel.

"This is your opportunity to send a message to these swindlers, these cold-blooded liars. I beg you, my friends. Don't send them back into the world with your blessing, but rather send them back into the streets with a sound thrashing they will never forget." He paused and flashed a smile. "I thank you for your kind consideration."

What an incredible crock of deceptive garbage. I felt nauseated. Nothern had given a brilliant summation—a stunning delivery by a man possessing an uncanny ability to almost caress the jury in his arms. This was a master attorney, and I knew I had just had my ass kicked.

What he said was nowhere close to the truth, but I conceded that he won the battle. I remembered the women's conversation I had overheard in the hallway and knew we were going to lose—and were going to lose big. I looked at Joseph Klockgether to check his reaction, which was pretty much the same as it had been through the trial. He looked at me with a slight smile on his face and shrugged.

It was now Winterbotham's turn to address the jury. I gave him a sideways glance, checking his mood and hoping his lithium was working.

He also warmly greeted the jury, thanking them for their kind attention. He said he hoped they would look at more than the excellent lawyering of Mr. Nothern's presentation, because this was not about calling me "the General," it was about facts.

"And the facts stack up fully on my client's side," he said. "The first point is that Mr. Harrington called Mr. Nelson. The most important issue of this entire case is whether this was a donation of the body and money to the CSC or a cloak-and-dagger clandestine business deal between Mr. Nelson and the Harrington brothers. If you find it was a donation, then of course you must find for the defendants, and that's why the plaintiffs have worked so hard to obscure that legal foundation by calling it a business deal. You swore an oath, and your responsibility requires that you confirm a legal judgment, not pass judgment on Mr. Nelson's beliefs.

"On the Harrington side we have their word, no evidence. On Mr. Nelson's side we have his word and documents signed by both the Harrington brothers. We also have the history of the CSC and CSNY, as well as CS Michigan's policy of refusing to accept a cryonic suspension without the body being donated to the society research program. With every freezing performed in the United States, there has never been a cryonic suspension without a donation of the body—including, I might add, this one."

I looked at the jury, hoping that Winterbotham was undoing some of Nothern's damage, but their faces were inscrutable. "It would be insane to do otherwise—you could be sued for it. We then examine the years of service donated by Mr. Nelson without salary or payment of any sort. He is a true believer, and it is not unusual to find true believers who spend their entire life fighting for their cause.

"You have seen where Mr. Nelson froze a number of friends and strangers at his own expense and took personal responsibility for their freezing for as long as he possibly could. We have seen where Mr. Nelson has given countless radio and television interviews, as well as lectures at colleges, hospitals, and national conferences.

"Mr. Nelson, along with the scientists and doctors he assembled, froze the world's first human being, Dr. James Bedford, on January 12, 1967. He wrote a book about cryonics and the freezing of Dr. Bedford. He built the world's first long-term storage vault on cemetery grounds, and he maintained several suspended cryonics patients by himself for years.

"What more can you ask of him? Was he sincere? You're damn right he was sincere. He gave this work his entire life and lost his wife and family because of his devout faith in cryonics."

Winterbotham paused and leaned against the jury box. He stopped for so long, I worried he had fallen asleep again. "He accepts the responsibility for the accidental failure and the loss of Mrs. Harrington, Genevieve de la Poterie, and Steven Mandell. Have you noticed that no one else is suing over the other patients lost in that same capsule, not Pauline Mandell or the de la Poterie family? They know Mr. Nelson gave it a 100 percent effort. And the biggest evidence of Mr. Nelson's character is his response to the capsule failure. He could have just hid it and not told anyone. Who would have known? He could have filled the capsule up with liquid nitrogen and pretended as if nothing had happened.

"That's what Mr. de la Poterie and Terry Harrington suggested. Just fill it up again and carry on as though it never happened. Mr. Nelson flew, at his own expense, to look Mr. de la Poterie and Mr. Harrington in the eye and explain the loss of the capsule. He then flew to Michigan and told the father of the cryonics movement, Professor Robert Ettinger, that there had been a failure at the cryonics facility.

"Without a doubt some mistakes were made, but, ladies and gentlemen, when you look at the enormity of Mr. Nelson's challenge, how could there not be setbacks? Mr. Nelson went to Iowa at Mr. Harrington's request and made the arrangements for placing Mrs. Harrington in suspension. He had the brothers sign all the proper legal forms for a donation, and here they are."

Winterbotham pointed at Terry Harrington, who immediately looked wide-eyed and innocent. "They claim they don't remember what they signed. It was enormously difficult to complete a suspension in Iowa; Mr. Nelson made that happen. And Mr. Nelson did not get the ten thousand dollars personally. That money was a donation to the CSC. Just look at the Harringtons' tax returns and I guarantee they show that both brothers took that ten thousand dollars as a tax deduction.

"The CSC kept Mrs. Harrington in temporary storage for two and a half years and then made it possible for the Harrington brothers to conduct a service and a two-hour viewing. This is no General, my friends; this is no man masquerading as Jesus Christ. This is a man who became caught up in something so big, it was like a tornado, and it threw him and his frozen friends through a storm.

"I think we must recognize that Bob Nelson picked up the cryo-ball and ran a long way with it. In some ways he made a touchdown, and in other ways he didn't. But one thing he never did was to make a secret deal outside of the cryonics circle with Terry and Dennis Harrington. That is why the ten-thousand-dollar check was sent to CSC offices and deposited into the CSC bank account. That money was used for dry ice replacement over the next thirty months.

"The total cost of the dry ice replacement over that time span was exactly $10,800, not counting the labor and the transport of one hundred miles per week. If you calculate that, it comes to twelve thousand miles of Mr. Nelson driving to faithfully replace that dry ice without ever missing once. Does that sound like a con man?

"I ask you to please be fair with Mr. Nelson. While you may not like the idea of frozen bodies and trying to bring people back from the dead, the ultimate truth is this: Was this transaction a donation, or was it a scam? I thank you sincerely for your honest consideration."

It was 11:30 a.m. when the judge dismissed the jury for lunch and ordered them back the next day for deliberations. Winterbotham and I arrived at about noon the following day and waited around. I kept asking him what he thought the jury would do, based on his experience and their expressions and demeanor. He shrugged and said it could go either way. At 3:00 p.m. the light went on in the courtroom, indicating that the jurors had reached a verdict. The verdict would be announced at 3:30.

I felt sick about Joseph Klockgether. He always had good intentions, but I feared that Nothern's angle of pitting Joseph and me as competition to God was going to be a tough hurdle to overcome. At 3:30 we were all standing at attention, facing the jury. The courtroom was packed with spectators and news media. My heart was racing, and I had to keep my hand on my knee to keep it from shaking. The court clerk asked in a loud, booming voice, "Ladies and gentlemen, have you reached a verdict?"

The forelady answered, "Yes we have."

"Would you please read the verdict?"

The forelady read loudly into a microphone. "On the matter of intentional infliction of emotional distress, we find as to the defendant Joseph Klockgether *for the plaintiffs*, Terry and Dennis Harrington, and order the defendant *to pay damages* in the amount of . . ."

With those words, it seemed like the building began to shake violently, accompanied by the roar of an enormous ocean tsunami. In my head I screamed, *No, no! You can't do this to this innocent wonderful man. Joe Klockgether only gave his help freely to those who asked for it. How could you not see this truth?*

A surge of rage and hurt rushed through my body like I had never felt before. I tuned out hearing the amount of the damages against Joseph Klockgether. I knew the same fate was about to fall on me, but I didn't care about myself. All I had was enough money for gas to get home!

I said as loud as I could, "You have no idea the mistake you have just made."

The forelady ignored me and continued rattling on with the judgment against Joseph. I was devastated for him. I stood up, walked past the jury, and stomped out of the courtroom. I was not giving them the pleasure of witnessing my reaction as they delivered the verdict against me.

My unexpected maneuver allowed me to avoid the ten news cameramen who were waiting to learn the verdict; they were caught completely unprepared for my sudden departure. I just rushed past them and their bewildered looks. I was almost out of the courthouse before they realized I was their story. They hollered, "Mr. Nelson, where are you-u-u-u . . ." as the Hall of Justice doors slammed shut behind me.

I had driven a friend's car to court that day since I didn't want to be with Winterbotham in case the verdict went against me. About halfway home I heard on the radio that Klockgether and I had been found at fault. *Four hundred thousand dollars . . . each.*

I slammed the off button on the radio, slammed the car door when I reached my apartment, and then slammed my bedroom door, those words reverberating inside my thick skull for hours.

I could feel the compassion, cultivated by my cryonics goals, draining from my body. My lifelong dream had resulted in catastrophe. I locked myself in my room for two days, needing to recover from getting my head smashed with a sledgehammer. Judgment day will endure forever as an excruciating memory—even if I am suspended and revived centuries in the future.

I now owed those vultures almost half a million dollars. I needed a new attorney, and it would cost twelve thousand dollars to obtain a copy of the transcript so that I could file an appeal. I vowed that day that I would never again discuss cryonics with anyone, beyond what might still be necessary to finish up this legal mess. I would forever turn off that cryonics switch in my head and once again make my children, who had for so many years seen so little of me, my focus for the rest of my life.

CHAPTER 16

Appeal and Settlement

THE INSULT OF THAT JURY'S DECISION WAS MORE THAN my soul and spirit could bear. I had given years of my life to this journey and had been condemned for my trouble. I tried hard to fight off the self-pity, but I still could not comprehend that this nightmare was the end product of all my hopes and dreams.

I was numb with disbelief at the verdict; the jury had ignored the facts and documentation and instead handed down an emotional verdict based on the image that Nothern had projected onto Klockgether and me.

The jury likely felt it was their job to stamp out a perceived assault on Christianity. It was, without a doubt, the prime objective of the plaintiffs' effort to pit us against God. That malevolent and hypocritical distortion made me sick. I had the deepest respect and love for the teachings of Christ; to me cryonics was a gift of the Creator, no different than organ transplants or any other heroic medical treatment.

My anger at these circumstances was almost unbearable. Joseph Klockgether, who had given his time and services free of charge for years, was also now expected to pay almost half a million dollars to these liars. If anyone had a right to hate me, it was Joseph. I had gotten him dragged into this trial, and I had made all the decisions that led to the closure of the vault. But the bloodsucking, soul-killing plaintiffs needed *me* to get at *Joseph's* insurance money. Despite everything, Joseph and I are friends to this day, as close as we were during the beginning days of the cryonics movement.

My friend Stella Gramer advised me to either appeal the verdict or move to Canada. "You can't avoid a punitive damage judgment; you can't even use bankruptcy against it. You have to appeal. There's simply no choice."

Between the judge not allowing the AGA documents and my lawyer's failure to disclose his lithium medication and his resulting crazy behavior in the courtroom, I had an excellent shot at winning an appeal. The only problem: I was flat broke. I had already sold my beloved Porsche to pay Winterbotham. There was nothing left.

I was grateful when my friend Sandra Stanley offered to help with my legal woes. She was a newly practicing attorney and immediately filed for the right to appeal with the second appellate court. Joseph's attorneys also filed. Sandra petitioned the court to waive the twelve-thousand-dollar fee for the trial transcript, basically telling them I was destitute. This was crucial to what happened later, and that snake Worthington watched closely.

I finally learned the loophole that justified the judge's inexplicable decision to exclude the Anatomical Gift Act. Judge Shelby had written the California attorney general before the trial and asked that if the AGA was fraudulently utilized, did that protect the person perpetuating the fraud? In a fit of bureaucratic sleight of hand, the reply stated that even if an organization was declared a medical research nonprofit, it didn't mean they actually were a medical research nonprofit. To my knowledge, there was never a hearing prior to Judge Shelby's ruling so that we could establish that the CSC was a legitimate foundation and we had not fraudulently used the AGA.

If I obtained the waiver, nothing would prevent a second trial. With Sandra's help, I could represent myself in court. A delicious benefit would be the nightmare I'd create for Worthington. Not only would the judgment against Joseph Klockgether's insurance company be delayed indefinitely, there was a real chance that Worthington could lose that judgment. However, without the waiver, I couldn't get my hands on the court transcripts, and no transcript meant no appeal.

About a month into the legal process, Sandra received a call from Nothern with an unexpected offer to settle the judgment against me.

Joseph's insurance company had made overtures, suggesting they would pay the debt, but they wanted to wait until my appeal was resolved. Nothern and the rest of the vultures needed my appeal dismissed so that they could get their hands on the four hundred thousand dollars in insurance money—the big prize. They knew I didn't have any money.

Their strategy proved very well thought out. Additionally, they wanted to represent me in a lawsuit against my attorney, Winterbotham. Of course they would pocket whatever money they managed to get from him.

I was now in the peculiar position of negotiating with the vermin and charlatans who had created this situation, destroyed my legacy in cryonics, and excoriated my honor in court. However, the offer sounded great. They could feast on Winterbotham if they dropped that ridiculous judgment against me. I just wanted to be freed of the ordeal, but I would reject the offer if it harmed Joseph.

I called Joseph the next morning and explained Nothern's offer. The trial's negative publicity had damaged his reputation, and a lien had been placed against his mortuary until the insurance company paid the judgment. My heart ached for him.

Joseph agreed to the offer and wanted to talk to his attorney. A couple days later, he called me back and said, "Don't be concerned about my case. Just do whatever you need to end this and put this insanity behind you."

This was a great relief. "Joe, I'm so sorry. I never thought we'd get to this point."

"Don't feel guilty on my account. I know this was a money grab, and I know there'll always be people like that. After all my years in the business, nothing surprises me."

I didn't feel charitable like Joseph. "Worthington surprised me. I'd heard about such nasty lawyers but had never met one. He engineered this whole thing—found the Harringtons, convinced them to sue, and fed them the lies." About that time I learned, too late unfortunately, that if I hadn't shown up for trial, Joseph would have won by default—there was no evidence against him. By trying to do the right thing morally, I did the worst thing possible strategically.

"For them it's just business," Joseph said. "That doesn't make it okay; it's just the way of the world."

Sandra and I made an appointment to meet with Nothern at his Century City office to finalize the agreement. I told Nothern that I would deal with him only and not with Worthington; that man had become the only person on this planet I actually hated. For me, *he* was the con artist, swindling an eight-hundred-thousand-dollar judgment out of the jury.

When we met, I told myself to smile, but I hated shaking Nothern's hand.

He patted my hand, his voice sounding as smooth as a hypnotist's. "Mr. Nelson, I'm so sorry for everything you've just gone through. I know this has been terribly difficult, but it will all be over soon."

With his instinct for knowing exactly what to say and how to say it, he had managed to enchant me once more. Sitting at that oak conference table in a sumptuous leather chair, sipping divine coffee that a gorgeous secretary had brought me, I felt like I was making some Faustian agreement. Although the deal was technically good, I still cringed at the injustice, since I had tried to help the plaintiffs. Through that verdict, I feared the lawyers' lies would become the official version of my actions at Chatsworth and negate my contributions to cryonics. After all my years of investing my time, my soul, and my money, I wondered what my lasting contribution to cryonics would be. In the end, had I advanced the goals that I loved? Had I helped advance the life's work of my hero, Professor Robert Ettinger? *Had my work mattered at all?*

My pen hovered over the settlement papers with the same trepidation I had felt when I sat in another lawyer's office and had signed my divorce papers. With that signature, I had ended my vow of lifelong commitment to my wife Elaine, and I knew these settlement papers would be my last act as a cryonicist. With this signature, all those hopes and dreams I had carried for more than fifteen years would fade into the past, becoming more hazy and irrelevant with each passing year. My life, which had once seemed so destined and sure, now seemed hazy, as though I was peering through the fog of liquid nitrogen vapor. I wondered about that man, that future Bob Nelson, who wasn't a cryonicist.

I was just about to sign the document when Nothern dropped what he tried to represent as a minor detail. Marie Brown wasn't willing to settle, so this agreement excluded her; that left me still owing her sixty-five thousand dollars. I stood up and paced the room in disgust—even now, there was more deception and more greed from these people. Sandra quickly reminded Nothern that the agreement was the dismissal of the entire judgment, which included Brown. This last-minute change was not acceptable; we left, papers unsigned. That tiny victory gave me a microscopic measure of happiness. The lawyer's charm hadn't worked this time.

Nothern eventually talked Brown into accepting the settlement, and I finally agreed as well. He also sued my attorney, Winterbotham, for me and received sixty thousand dollars; I got nothing. While I waited on the settlement, the court extended the deadline to file briefings. Sandra never filed, and we allowed the appeal to die on the vine. On January 25, 1983, the following judgment was handed down: "Pursuant to appellant Robert F. Nelson's request, the appeal is dismissed." It was over.

With the signing of the settlement papers, I banished cryonics from my mind and heart forever. All my love and passion was gone, robbed from me in a courtroom by people who cared only about pilfering a buck.

CHAPTER 17

Closed Doors, Opened Windows

I HAD ONE ASSET LEFT—MY ELECTRONICS REPAIR BUSINESS, California Video Repair, in Huntington Beach. At least I could sleep and eat in the back of the store. After suffering an almost lethal blow to my soul, I reverted from using my biological father's name back to my stepdad's name, Robert Buccelli. I simply wanted *Bob Nelson* to disappear. Whenever I received any requests for an interview, I hung up the phone without saying a word. Bob Nelson was on another planet.

Slowly I crawled back into the world of the living. I found a home in Huntington Beach and started life over again. For the next three years, I worked at my repair business day and night. All the energy that I had invested in the vault now went into the store.

It wasn't until 1987 that I recovered from the cryonics fiasco. I went home one evening and cooked myself a big filet mignon. With a glass of fine red wine, I retired to my backyard to watch a gorgeous mountain sunset. I thought, *Wow, I am pretty lucky. I've got it all.* Then I heard a voice taunting me: "Is this really it Bob—a big steak, a new Honda Prelude, a nice home? Are you *really* happy now?"

I knew almost at once that I was kidding myself. I was missing one of the most important elements of being alive—that of being in love.

Several months later I was driving to my store in Huntington Beach. Just before the freeway entrance stood a bakery where I occasionally stopped for coffee and blueberry muffins.

As I entered the bakery, I noticed a breathtaking Asian woman working the counter. She was a petite, smiling beauty with silken black hair to her knees. After gazing too long at her, I managed to say, "Hello."

I ordered my coffee and muffin. All week, I couldn't stop thinking of this beautiful lady who glowed with an enormous inner radiance. She certainly had attracted my attention. Though not worldly, her eyes revealed a startling awareness that was utterly enchanting.

I stopped in the bakery every morning, but I was making zero progress. I learned that her name was Moeurth and she was thirty-three. She had emigrated from Cambodia and had lived in the United States for five years. After the first week, I invited her to lunch at a restaurant a block away. She said no and explained that she had never been on a date. In her country, her father picked her husband, and she was not yet ready.

By the second week I was becoming frustrated. She always waited on me with a big smile, remembered my order, and asked me sweetly, "How are you today? You go to work?" However, I couldn't make the slightest progress, so I decided to appeal to her younger sister for help. Penny also worked at the bakery, was more Americanized, and was excited to play matchmaker. In the third week, Moeurth handed me a bag with two blueberry muffins instead of my usual one.

She gave me a shy smile and said, "The other is for your wife."

I was thrilled she thought of me. "I'm not married, ma'am. I'm too young." We both just smiled—very warm smiles. It was a good day.

The next day Penny told me that Moeurth had agreed to lunch, but she would drive her own car the two hundred yards to the restaurant.

I thought it was strange but was happy with whatever I could get. At lunch she ordered only a Coke.

"How can I become your friend?" I asked.

"That is my parents' decision," she replied.

"How can your parents consider me if we haven't met?"

"I don't know, but I will ask them."

Two days later, Moeurth said her parents had invited me to their home in Pomona. I was excited; this quest was like climbing a mountain, but I was doing it.

When I arrived at her home, I saw that it contained many small rugs and several lovely, colorful sheets hung from the ceiling to partition off different parts of the rooms for privacy. Her mom greeted me with some kind Cambodian words and then handed me a huge bowl of fruit and gestured for me to sit on a worn-out couch. Her mom and I exchanged big smiles and a few words during my two-hour visit. When I used the bathroom, I counted thirteen toothbrushes. This was truly a loving family, struggling to keep their way of life intact.

The next week I met her father at the Pomona Buddhist temple, where he was serving a six-month commitment as a monk. The temple was a converted three-bedroom house, retrofitted with stained-glass windows and gold-plated steel horns on the four corners of the roof. Orange and yellow rugs covered the floor of the spartan room, and pictures of great monks and mountains adorned the walls. The four Cambodian monks wore ochre robes over one shoulder, and they all had shaved heads. I felt quite honored and nervous when they welcomed me, but I quickly felt their acceptance.

Her father gave his permission for our first date at Knotts Berry Farm. After about two hours of blissful togetherness, I took a bold step and reached out to hold her hand. She was shy but didn't pull away and soon relaxed.

"I'm so happy to have this chance to take you out."

"This is very new for me and not at all the Cambodian way."

"Yes, but you're in America now. You are now both Cambodian and American, so you need to learn how to integrate this exciting new world into your precious life."

Moeurth nodded. When things were explained logically, I realized that she and her family were quite willing to adapt.

Against her wishes, I bought her a jacket. She was confused about how to handle the difference in cultures, while I tried to be sensitive to this strain on her conscience. I was falling in love.

On our third date, as we ate a meal of fish and clams, Moeurth said, "Bob, I need tell something important." In her beautiful broken English, she told me that after three dates, we couldn't see each other again.

She explained that Cambodians do not allow any more connection without an engagement agreement. I sat there stunned. I wasn't thinking about engagement; we'd only just started dating. I balked at the all-or-nothing prospect, but I was scared to lose her entirely.

When I brought her home before dark, Moeurth said, "Not to worry about us. We enjoyed each other's company. Thank you so much for our wonderful friendship."

No hug, no kiss, not even a handshake, just good-bye. She closed the door, and then she was gone forever. I stood outside, staring up at her house, and wondered if this supposed Cambodian custom was merely a pretense for breaking off our relationship. *Had I been in love alone?*

On my drive home, I gripped the steering wheel and tried to console myself by thinking I would simply move on to the next woman. I wasn't a bad catch, I thought. But Moeurth had morals and honor such as I had never before encountered. And my heart would not listen to this "other woman" nonsense; it knew whom I loved. Each morning I drove by her bakery, and I felt a painful longing to call her.

Still reeling from the lies and duplicity of the trial, I was attracted to her genuine and innocent heart. I knew she wasn't a delicate child; her life hadn't been sheltered. Moeurth had been a happy girl in Cambodia. They never had electricity or running water, but they had a cow she doted on, and her father carved her any toy she wanted from wood. As a teenager, though, she had been placed in a Communist prison camp and forced to work in the rice fields every waking hour for three and a half years. Guarded by soldiers dressed all in black with machine guns on horseback, she witnessed them executing her friends and family by slashing their throats or bellies with their long knives. But through all her hardships, she had maintained her serenity and sweetness. I had become cynical after the cryonics trial, but Moeurth had never lost her optimism and never would. She would have been an amazing wife.

Two weeks later, when I could not endure her absence any longer, I called her and asked, "Moeurth, can we meet to talk about engagement?"

After a pause she said, "I must speak to my parents. They must give their permission if we are to talk about marriage."

I was shocked at the string of difficulties. With cryonics, I had wanted to take a time machine into the future. With Moeurth, it felt like I was taking a time machine into the past. It didn't matter though; I'd follow her anywhere. I asked, "What if they don't approve of our marriage?"

"Bob, I came into this world through the love of my precious parents. They are like God to me, and I have been taught to respect their guidance and wisdom. I will honor whatever they decide."

Moeurth called me the next day and explained her father's stipulations for the marriage. They would convene the entire family in two weeks for everyone to have an opportunity to meet and question this American. They would determine whether I was worthy of marrying their beloved Moeurth. Additionally, I needed to bring at least ten character witnesses who would speak for my character and sincerity in this engagement.

On the day of the examination, about forty Cambodian people came to Moeurth's house. One of Moeurth's brothers-in–law, Sarinn, sat the family on the front lawn in a circle with one chair in the center for me. Moeurth was beautifully dressed in a long golden gown, her knee-length jet-black hair piled on her head.

An elder Cambodian began the discussion by asking my supporters to introduce themselves and express what they felt about Bob Buccelli to the friends and family. After all their compliments, the attention turned to me.

"Will you join Moeurth's family or try to keep her unto yourself?"

"I have honestly grown to care for her family. It would be an extreme honor to be considered part of this family. I would love to learn and participate in your customs."

This seemed to please most, except for one gentleman who wanted to delve into my personal relationships and my ex-wife, who had been remarried for nearly ten years and had a daughter with her new husband.

Although I had expected difficult questions, I began to feel upset when another brother interrupted. "Bob, please don't get frustrated. We are just trying to be as careful as we possibly can. Moeurth is a grown woman, but we love her immensely and want her safe and happy. Please understand that."

One of the friendlier brothers asked, "Robert, why do you wish to marry a woman of another culture?"

I turned to look at Moeurth and paused to choose my words carefully. "She is a flower and more beautiful than words can describe. Inside I have found an even finer soul. I will treasure her all of my days."

With that came a round of applause and one last question. Because of the language difficulty, I thought they were asking when I wanted their decision. I said firmly, "I want that right now."

The entire group roared with laughter.

The leader explained, "We were asking when you would like to marry if the group approved—not when we would give our decision."

After dinner, Penny announced that the family would happily accept me as the husband of their precious Moeurth. "From this moment on until you become man and wife, you are both just like birds locked in a cage and waiting to be joined together. You are a lucky man, Robert."

Amid the cheering, I went to Moeurth, whom I was still not allowed to touch. For the first time I said, "I love you."

Now we could speak daily by phone or go out for a brief meal if the outing was related to our wedding plans.

The marriage could not occur until the dowry of five thousand dollars was paid to her father. Moeurth explained that usually an engaged couple would work together, sometimes for years, to save the money. She suggested that with us both working and saving, we could get married within a year or two. I told her, "I have the money, and I don't want to wait." Moeurth then asked me for one special favor; her mother wanted an authentic Cambodian ceremony, which lasted two days and required eight costume changes for me and ten for Moeurth.

I happily honored her mother's request, although I had no idea what it would entail. We were married on June 16, 1990. The celebration began at 9:00 a.m. on the fifteenth, and the first day ended at 6:00 p.m. The ceremony took place in the back of Moeurth's home. Thirty people filtered in throughout the day. Everyone in the family was busy cooking, preparing the next performance, and helping with the costume changes. Both days Moeurth and I kneeled on a dais and soaked in the spectacle. I couldn't understand the words or the reenacted symbolism, but our wedding was filled with a stunning pageantry of colorful rented costumes and professional dancers in golden sedge hats and surrounded by red and gold paper decorations. Moeurth wore a matchless gown of gold sequins that accentuated her long silken hair. No matter how much my knees ached during those long hours kneeling on the floor, one look at my angelic bride revitalized me. The music and the dancers were entrancing; at times I felt as though I had died and gone to heaven. The only thing missing was my children. They were invited of course, but their own problems prevented their attendance.

At the end of the first day ceremonies, I was absolutely exhausted and asked, "Are we married now?"

Moeurth's younger sister, Penny, answered, "No Robert, but we're getting close."

The second day was another marathon of singing, posing, and professional dancers. About noon, Penny rather unceremoniously hollered

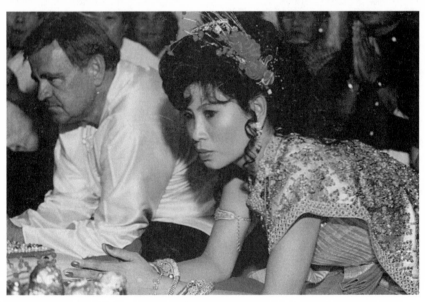

Giving thanks for another day of loving

across the room, "Bob, she's yours now." I will remember that sentence forever as one of life's finest.

At six o'clock on the second evening, we finished our Herculean wedding. This princess would be coming home with me. What a joy! That night we attended a ball in our honor with over three hundred people joining in the celebration of our union. It was a spectacular eight-course feast of fried rice with shrimp, vegetables, whole carp, soup, and a wider variety of fruit than a farmers' market.

It wasn't long before someone asked to see us kiss.

"Finally," I said, "we will share our first kiss." As I took her in my arms for the first time, I closed my eyes and readied myself. I was once again frustrated when my lips touched the side of her cheek. She had turned her head at the last second. Everyone at the table laughed hysterically at my disappointment.

People at the next table again asked to see us kiss; this time I put my hand under her chin and guided her lips to meet mine. Time stopped in that magical moment. It was done. We had made it all come true just like she wanted, and now my ravishing wife would come to our home.

Over the past twenty-two years, Moeurth and I have enjoyed a marriage of love and respect without a single fight. We have brought two wonderful half-Italian–half-Cambodian girls into the world. We have certainly had disagreements, but through our deep admiration, we have managed to resolve them with calm consideration for each other. Only once did we come close to angry words over parental control of our two daughters. After I strongly had my say, Moeurth looked at me with a tear rolling down her cheek and then walked away without saying a word. I of course was brought to my knees by that tear and profusely apologized.

There was one exception during my twenty-five-year hiatus from the world of cryonics. I had left the cryonics movement without offering any justification, so in 1991 I granted Mike Perry, historian for the Alcor Foundation, and his two associates a forty-five minute interview.

I had never mentioned my cryonics past to my wife, and I felt I owed her that explanation after we had been married one year. She was intrigued by my past but not bothered. Compared to surviving a Pol Pot concentration camp in Cambodia and adjusting to American life, my delay in revealing this bit of history seemed minor to her.

Cryonics was beyond Moeurth's ability to understand. She was confused and I dare say frightened by the concept. She had seen so much death in her life and couldn't comprehend how a person might possibly come back. She often said, "Honey, me no want freeze, OK?" I always chuckled under my breath and replied, "Okay, darling, don't worry; I won't freeze you."

Almost two decades later, I decided to write my story. Word had gotten to Sam Shaw, a producer for *This American Life*, and I agreed to an interview. Shortly afterward, Moeurth came to me and said, "Honey I have something to say. Please listen clearly. After many years of consideration and learning, now I want freeze. Now I understand."

CHAPTER 18

Ted Williams—
The Story of One Recent Suspension

WHEN NEWS BROKE THAT BELOVED BASEBALL PLAYER TED WILLIAMS had been cryonically preserved, I watched the Williamses' family drama unfold from the sidelines, still in self-imposed exile from cryonics. I was amazed by how far the technology had advanced in those years, yet the ensuing controversy was eerily familiar.

For more than thirty-five years, the cryonics movement had been hoping for famous individuals to choose cryopreservation. Prior to Ted Williams, perhaps the most famous cryopatient had been Richard "Dick Clair" Jones. Jones was a TV scriptwriter and producer for several shows, including *The Facts of Life, Flo*, and *Mama's Family*, and had won three Emmy awards for *The Carol Burnett Show*. Jones left some two million dollars to Alcor when he was cryopreserved in 1988. On July 5, 2002, Ted Williams was declared clinically dead and cryopreserved. As with so many other cryonic suspensions, controversy swirled around the case.

In 1996 Williams had signed a will stating that he wished to be cremated and his ashes scattered over the ocean off the Florida coast, where he'd been an avid fisherman. But his son, John-Henry, had become interested in cryonics. He had studied the literature and spoken with experts, and he wanted his famous father preserved in "biostasis"—cryopreserved—for possible later reanimation. As an indication of the love between father and son, Ted had given his son power of attorney over his estate. At that time, both John-Henry and his sister, Claudia, were named as beneficiaries in the will. A child of an earlier marriage, Barbara Joyce "Bobby Jo" Ferrell, had become estranged from her father and was excluded.

When Ted Williams was close to the end of his life, John-Henry called the Alcor Foundation from the Florida hospital. John-Henry requested that the Alcor recovery team come to Florida at once. A private airplane was on standby to fly Williams from Florida to Scottsdale. The operating room and surgical team at Alcor were on full alert, waiting for the patient's arrival. The private airport adjacent to the Alcor facility brought Williams's body to within a few minutes' drive of Alcor's front door.

As with all cryonic suspensions, rapid action is vital, and Alcor was ready. On July 5, 2002, at 2:10 p.m., the great Ted Williams's heart stopped beating and he was pronounced clinically dead. At once the Alcor team took over and introduced a cooling agent through the carotid artery, while a heart-massaging machine maintained Williams's heart at a normal rhythm. The objective was to reestablish circulation and cool the brain as fast as possible while lowering the entire body temperature.

His body was released by hospital officials and rushed by emergency medical vehicle to the waiting jet, which promptly headed for Arizona. As the plane landed in Scottsdale, the medical team prepared Williams for the transfer to the waiting ambulance, which soon delivered him to the Alcor operating room.

Once he was on the table, the medical team took over preparing the body, shaving his head and adjusting tubes and valves. After about thirty minutes of preparation, they began to surgically remove, or "isolate," the head, having first obtained John-Henry's approval. This step was controversial to many in cryonics, including Professor Ettinger, especially since this was a whole-body preservation, which some interpreted as an "*intact whole body*." The surgical isolation was intended to optimize perfusion or infusion of cryoprotectant into the brain via the neck arteries.

As the seat of consciousness, feeling, memory, and selfhood, the brain is the all-important part of the anatomy for future recovery of a person. By optimizing the cryoprotection of the brain, the doctors could achieve a new, high level of preservation known as vitrification. As the patient was cooled to cryogenic temperatures, vitrification would prevent the formation of damaging ice crystals as cooling progressed. In this way, the quality of preservation is greatly improved over earlier techniques, further raising hopes that eventually the patient can be recovered in a healthy state. Such recovery would involve treating any ailments, including aging, and of course reattaching the head to the rest of the preserved body with all connections of blood vessels, nerves, and other structures restored.

At the time, cryopreservation techniques did not permit vitrification of the whole body, so the rest of the body, or trunk, was perfused by another method, and both head and trunk were cooled to cryogenic temperatures. For a while the head was stored at about -130°C in a low-temperature refrigeration unit known as the Cryostar, and then both head and body were transferred to an upright capsule and submerged in liquid nitrogen.

Controversy boiled up even as Ted Williams was undergoing the careful preparations at Alcor. Bobby Jo, the estranged daughter, insisted that her father be cremated as requested in his 1996 will. Meanwhile, John-Henry produced a document he had retrieved from the trunk of his car dated November 2, 2000, and signed by himself; his father, Ted; and his sister, Claudia. The note indicated their agreement "to be put into Bio-Stasis after we die. This is what we want, to be able to be together in the future, even if it is only a chance." The document, if proven genuine, would supersede the request in the will for cremation. Two different testing labs determined the signature of Ted Williams to be genuine. The analysis also determined that Ted and John-Henry used the same pen, while Claudia used a different one. Claudia testified in a sworn affidavit to the note's authenticity.

Regardless of these results, Bobby Jo claimed the note was a forgery and did not negate the cremation request. She agreed to accede to her father's wishes in exchange for a settlement from the estate amounting to several hundred thousand dollars. Ted Williams remains in suspension and was joined at Alcor by his son when he died of leukemia in 2004.

Ted Williams's procedure of a whole body suspension should not be confused with another option as a final effort to save the patient: to recover only the head and allow the rest of the body to go. The rationale is that the brain is the important part and that head-only, or "neuro," preservation might be sufficient to recover the entire patient someday, when the rest of the body could be replaced by advanced means of tissue and organ regeneration. Preserving just the head would save greatly on maintenance expenses and might have made it possible to stretch CSC's meager funds enough that some or all of the suspensions could have been continued.

I learned much later that Ev Cooper had written about neuro-preservation (head only) in the 1960s, but it was not much considered, if at all, in the early years. The idea of decapitation is morbid and profoundly associated with the very worst of circumstances; of course people didn't want to think about it. If they did consider it, people questioned whether the body could be replaced as hoped, whether the result would still be the original person, and so on. I don't remember that neuro-preservation was ever discussed until after the capsule failures, when it was too late. If we had, I shudder to think how Nothern would have exploited decapitation at our trial. No one was neuro-preserved before Alcor's first suspension in July 1976, and the practice is still controversial. None of those I froze had expressed a wish for a neuro option, or to be converted to it should the funds run short. None of the relatives told me they wanted it performed as a way of either reducing expenses for their loved ones or continuing a suspension if it otherwise had to be terminated. During my years of involvement, we never tried or even considered the head-only option.

The struggle among Ted's children over what evidently amounted to money proved stressful to those in cryonics, because the procedures designed for optimum care seemed morbid to the public. In addition to the head being isolated, the skull was drilled with small openings, or burr holes, to observe the brain during the perfusion process. During the later cool-down to cryogenic temperatures, an apparatus detected sound bursts, indicating small hairline cracks formed in the solidified tissue, as normally occurred. These cracks too must be repaired by future technology, but in terms of loss of information, they are believed to be quite minor. Larry Johnson, an Alcor employee, leaked confidential information to the media in violation of the wishes of John-Henry and Claudia. A legislative initiative was started to restrict or eliminate cryonics in Arizona. In the end, this effort failed, and things returned to normal as media attention subsided. Cryonics in Arizona and elsewhere continues much as before. The wry observation was made that perhaps one day Ted Williams can confirm his real wishes and whether he is satisfied with how things finally turned out.

As of July 2013, numerous celebrities and millionaires have made covert arrangements for themselves. There are about 250 people currently in suspended animation; and well over a thousand people like you and me are all signed up, waiting for a time capsule ride into the future.

When we consider how far the science of human suspended animation has already advanced, we have vast reason to embrace a sublime, greatly extended life on the beautiful planet we call Earth.

CHAPTER 19

The Conclusion

The underlying Reality has cloaked itself in the cease-
lessly transforming cosmos, declaring itself without
revealing itself. The purpose of each soul's sojourn on
earth is to learn to see beyond the evanescence of phe-
nomena to the Eternal Reality.
                    —PARAMAHANSA YOGANANDA

BY FAR THIS IS THE MOST EXCITING CHAPTER TO WRITE. Why? For me
the conclusion is really the beginning. In fact, the entire goal of cryonics is
to delay any ending by hundreds of years. Thinking back on my epic near-
fifty-year cryonics journey, I can honestly say most of it was an honor and
only a small part of it was a nightmare.

As a devoted advocate of cryonics during that heady ten-year period,
I was president of the Cryonics Society of California and seized the
opportunity to freeze the first man, first woman, and first child. As one
of the movement's most prolific spokesmen, I taught people about this
optimistic new science in numerous interviews and TV shows, including
interviews with Regis Philbin and Phil Donohue. Through those years, I
had an incredible journey.

Dr. Bedford has been suspended for more than forty-five years, and
he is still only minutes into the dying process. If all goes well, he will
remain in this stage of early clinical death for centuries if need be, until
science determines his fate. Even if there is no hope for this man, he has
taken the first step in humanity's search for extended life. It was easy for

later cryonics activists to criticize our actions in those first days. During Dr. Bedford's suspension, we did not have a cooperating mortuary or even a sympathetic mortician.

The story of Dr. Bedford's freezing appeared in the first six pages of *Life* magazine's February 3, 1967, issue. I was excited about the potential exposure. An interesting but unfortunate aside is that for only the second time in its history, after two million copies of the issue had been printed and mailed to subscribers, *Life* stopped the presses. The first nine pages were replaced with the story of Grissom, White, and Chaffee, the three *Apollo 1* astronauts who died when their capsule caught fire during a pre-launch test. Consequently, our article was scrapped. The only other time *Life* axed a story was after the Kennedy assassination.

I had first become interested in cryonics because I knew that suspended animation was the best way to make long-distance spaceflight possible. I mourned the loss of those astronauts and pioneers, and yet I was confident that unfortunate tragedy and failure would not prevent future manned spaceflight. On the now-retired launchpad where the *Apollo 1* explosion occurred, one of the memorial plaques states:

> *In memory of those who made the ultimate sacrifice*
> *so others could reach for the stars;*
> Ad astra per aspera
> *(A rough road leads to the stars)*

The next ten years did not proceed like that early success; instead I spent them like I was hanging on to the side of a mountain by my fingernails. I had dedicated myself to making cryonic suspension available to Americans at the end of their life. However, my great project suffered a long, slow death. After acquiring nine—and losing seven—frozen bodies, I had to give up.

After losing my friends and after my abject failure with the vault, the lawsuits that recast my motives in the worst possible way were a devastating sucker punch. With such horrendous charges being made against Joseph Klockgether and me, everyone involved with cryonics might have run and hidden. With the exception of the CSC's secretary, Paul Porcasi, who feared his name being mentioned, every other officer, friend, and neighbor of the Cryonics Society voluntarily took the stand on our behalf. A few years later I received some sense of justice when that snake Worthington was disbarred, partly because of my case.

I spent the next twenty-five years in self-imposed exile from cryonics. I was largely silent and allowed other people to castigate and vilify me, fairly or not, as creating a "black stain" on cryonics. I haven't told my full story to correct history . . . until here and now.

But God chose differently, and this story did not end on such a sour note. I kept my promise for twenty-five years, staying largely silent as other people rewrote the history of what happened at the Chatsworth cemetery, and unfortunately I gave unspoken credence to the horrendous judgment against me. Today the cemetery owners deny they ever heard of cryonics and that a cryonics vault was ever built there. However, the location is still visible, and currently at least seven people are interred in the CSC underground vault there.

Eventually I came out of my self-induced coma to once again embrace cryonics. I was close to retirement and itching to write this book, mostly for my children. I called Professor Ettinger, and he gave his approval, saying, "I always know where your heart is."

After those years, I've acquired some perspective on CSC's contributions to cryonics. We propelled the cause forward by years when we froze Dr. Bedford. The CSC was the first to implement the Anatomical Gift Act, which is still used by cryonics organizations today. Even our failures, as with all young sciences, had beneficial effects by illustrating mistakes to be avoided in the future.

This subject has always been sensational and attracted high demand for debate and conflict. Many conservative scientists today believe that reanimation will never succeed. However, I prefer to focus on tomorrow's anticipated achievements rather than the limited means of today. Of course we realize it is not possible now to reanimate a frozen human—the consideration is about tomorrow!

Today I know differently from my beliefs during those invigorating days of early optimism. Just as the science evolves, so too must our human perceptions for scientific breakthroughs to succeed. Advance any controversial theory that attracts the attention of the popular media or religious leaders and isn't fully proven, and most scientists or the bureaucratic infrastructure will inundate the pioneers with reasons it will never work. Science, like nascent countries and philosophies, needs cowboys and revolutionaries, but unfortunately the rigors of the scientific method, while certainly necessary, can squelch discovery before it advances from hypothesis to experiment.

The truth is, no one can say with certainty what the future will bring. The distant future of one or two centuries *cannot be known* by anyone alive today! A cave dweller might well say "Man can never fly," but it takes people of vision to see beyond the darkness of their cave. Men whose vision we take for granted, such as Arthur C. Clarke, said cryonic suspension will someday be just another choice of interment.

⊷

In 2004 I received an invitation to visit the Alcor cryonics facility in Scottsdale, Arizona, and I visited my old friend, Dr. James Bedford. I was in awe of Alcor and what they had accomplished since I had walked away from cryonics in 1981. The management treated me like royalty, and I was deeply honored. When I was shown Dr. Bedford's capsule, I embraced it. Thirty-seven years had passed since I had last seen him, and this was an emotional reunion.

The next year, I was tentatively reentering the cryonics world while visiting the state-of-the-art cryonic storage facilities at the Cryonics Institute in Clinton Township, Michigan. I was happy to talk with the former CSNY president, Curtis Henderson, at the home of Professor Ettinger. We hadn't seen each other for twenty years. Curtis was gracious, but I could sense that he had some passion in his heart, and I encouraged him to spit it out. That was the reason I had traveled to this meeting. I thought to myself, *If anyone wants to say something or ask me something— say it to my face. Here I am, let it be now.*

Curtis told me that I had undermined the cryonics movement. He said that once a leader of a cryonics group had accepted responsibility for suspending patients, he had a sacred duty to allow nothing to get in the way of keeping those patients in suspension forever. There was absolutely no acceptable excuse for not doing so, none whatsoever.

When he finished, I asked him, "If what you said is true, then can you please explain the suspension patients at the CSNY facility? They eventually had the same fate as every CSC patient—being buried or cremated."

Curtis looked at me as though I had just hit him in the head with a baseball bat. He sat staring at me, not saying a word, thinking I know not what.

After a good fifteen minutes of just staring at me, he got up and went into his bedroom. I was unsure what was going to happen. Curtis reappeared a half hour later, and we spent the next couple of days being very cordial and respectful to each other. He was a true pioneer, trying to keep

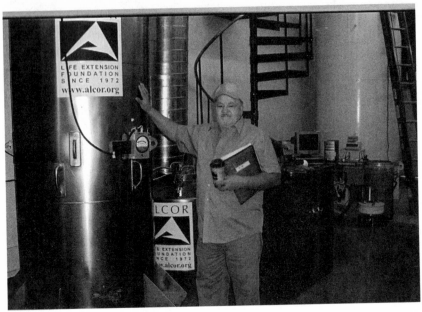

Bob Nelson stands next to the dewar containing Dr. James Bedford.

the patients at his New York facility in suspension. We did the very best with what we had; however, we both reached a point when *without money* we could go no further.

On my last visit to the Michigan facility, after I had completed all my legal and financial arrangements for my own cryonic suspension, I was privileged to witness an unforgettable moment in the main storage area where ten huge cryogenic capsules are under twenty-four-hour surveillance, each holding eight patients in liquid nitrogen.

In this room full of enormous, pure-white, human cryogenic containers stood a petite, lovely lady named Bridgett. She walked up to one of these gigantic vessels, placed her face on the resin-fiberglass with her arms outstretched, hugging the enormous unit, and said, "I'm here, darling, and I'll join you when my time comes. Please know that I love you with all my heart!"

With everything said and done, I stand before the world and future generations with a clear conscience and an open heart. I accept my lumps for my dumb mistakes. To the best of my recollection, this is exactly how it happened. And my sole purpose for writing this book is to leave a sincere accounting of my journey.

As Dr. Bedford told me the day before his body was frozen more than forty-five years ago, I repeat here today: If I am never to be resuscitated, I do this so my children and grandchildren might participate in the wonders of science and future medicine.

One summer day in July 2011, I was struck by an odd sense of foreboding and phoned Professor Ettinger. I eventually reached a nurse who told me he was in a coma and near clinical death. I pleaded with her to let me know if he regained consciousness. Two years earlier, after my *This American Life* interview, I had been approached by Hollywood producers and directors about filming my life story. I had just heard some exciting news about the cryonics movie and wanted Professor Ettinger to know. The actors had been chosen, and the film's production seemed assured. After his death, I received this e-mail from his daughter-in-law.

Bob was made aware, in his final hours, of your call and of the impend-
ing movie, which made him smile, very possibly his last smile. He was a
brave, brilliant visionary. He got the best suspension that preparation,
attention to detail, and love could get him. If there is a sequel to this life,
I'm sure he will be in it.

Connie Ettinger

I am now seventy-six years old and a lot closer to death than when I first read Professor Ettinger's book; my place is secured at Cryonics Institute in Michigan. I don't fear my voyage to the Undiscovered Country. I know the infrastructure now exists to keep me suspended, and I have full confidence that future generations will keep pushing toward those unknown frontiers. I know that *they* will sooner or later answer all of today's questions, including the possibility of reviving a frozen human being. My journey isn't over yet—it's only just begun.

I now have two older daughters, Lori and Susan, with my first wife, Elaine, and two younger daughters; Natalie is seventeen and Christine is twenty-two. They are starting their own journey. I wonder about all the scientific miracles that will come to pass during their lifetime, once I'm gone and lying in stasis in liquid nitrogen. *What part will their generation play in advancing human hibernation and suspended animation? How many millions of lives will be saved?*

The conclusion really brings me back to the beginning—to years before and the original path I had chosen for CSC, which was finding a scientific advisory board that could lead to reliable suspended animation. It's astonishing how far I had drifted from that original course. My personal passion had always been to discover how to sustain astronauts in suspended animation for months or even years. For me the solution to our limited life span, and therefore our limited travel distance to the planets, rested with science and advanced thinkers such as Professor Ettinger,

Albert Einstein, and other visionaries. If scientists are unable to find a way to travel near the speed of light, then we must make the travel time irrelevant. One day we could send humans to explore throughout the solar system and beyond.

Such worlds are just waiting for us to discover their amazing and strange features, possibly even life. Beyond our solar system await planets, stars, and whole swarms of galaxies. Mastery of such prospects as human hibernation and suspended animation will catapult humanity to a kind of superman traveling the universe at will. And who wouldn't love to be Superman?

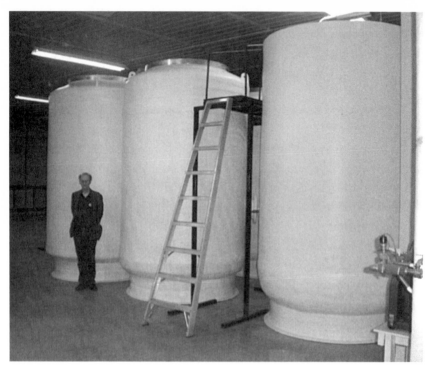

This is today's reality: 118 patients are frozen at this facility in hopes of future reanimation.

Epilogue

My story is now told, and I hand over the narrative of my personal experiences to the technology and astounding wonders of nature. The work of others shows all the potential and promise that has inspired me through the decades. For me, the Wright brothers' struggle to fly with man-made heavier-than-air craft has a special poignancy. Most of their contemporaries rejected the Wrights' experiments. The audacity of these mere bicycle mechanics, without even a high school diploma, thinking they could teach the world how to fly. Surely this must be a joke. It hadn't mattered that Leonardo da Vinci had left meticulous drawings on how such flying wings might one day be realized. On December 17, 1903, Orville made man's first flight at Kitty Hawk, North Carolina. Today there are at least ten methods of flight, including the NASA rocket plane, the Falcon HTV-2, which travels at thirteen thousand miles per hour—that's California to New York in fifteen minutes.

We have made astonishing progress since man has moved from the cave into the cosmos. Discoveries and enlightenment are happening faster and faster; I dare not project how life on earth will be in the coming centuries.

Looking around at today's advancements in medical technology, I see proof of the principle that "death" isn't final and that human hibernation is a reality. I feel at ease knowing that my efforts were not in vain. I'm always wondering, *What will be the world's next great scientific discovery?*

From the sidelines I've seen technology march on all around me—inexorably continuing with new medical miracles, both great and small. The examples I will offer here are just a trickle of what is quickly becoming an ocean of new intelligence. Mankind is on a roller-coaster ride into the heavens and the discovery of creation's purpose, which I believe will be complete enlightenment of the human mind and greatly extended, youthful life. Remember: Not so long ago, the world believed that if you sailed too far out onto the ocean, you would fall off!

INSPIRATION IN THE NATURAL WORLD

I've learned through the years of astonishing adaptations and feats of survival. We look to them as analogies of the possibilities that can be harnessed for humanity. One powerful lesson I've learned is that *life*, this inexplicable life force, always finds a way to endure.

During a heat or dry spell, the African lungfish undergoes estivation (triggered by heat instead of cold), a dormant state similar to hibernation. It can stay dormant for years, waiting for its environment to return to normal. The lungfish can remain in this deep sleep for up to five years.

In 1977 six-foot-long tube worms were discovered among an ecological system of hundreds of diverse life-forms, thousands of feet deep near 800°F ocean vents close to the island of Guam. These tube worms grow about one-half inch per year; some have lived as long as two hundred fifty years, making them among the longest-living animals known to science. And they live with absolutely no sun!

The water bear might be the toughest creature on the planet. This tiny animal, which looks like a microscopic caterpillar, can survive temperatures from a bitter -400°F to a hellish 300°F, tolerate a thousand times more radiation than other animals, and survive a decade without water. It is a breathtaking example of what is possible within the realm of living creatures.

Can any complete organism withstand immersion in liquid nitrogen? The nematode *Haemonchus contortus*, a parasite that infects goats, has survived several months of submersion in liquid nitrogen without preparation, damage, or negative results. Other life-forms can tolerate frozen suspension but require some treatment, such as a biological antifreeze.

The common mayfly lives for just one day and never eats. The giant California redwood lives several thousand years. At least one animal has actually achieved immortality. The captivating immortal jellyfish (*Turritopsis nutricula*) has somehow discovered the fountain of youth. This creature is able to cycle from a mature adult stage to an immature polyp and then back again and again.

NATURAL INSTANCES OF HUMAN HIBERNATION

Cryonics is not the only means of slowing down the biological clock in an effort to extend human life. In 1969 Armando Socarras Ramirez was a seventeen-year-old stowaway in a lower cargo compartment of a DC-8 plane bound for Madrid from Cuba. During the eight-hour flight, he was exposed to -30°F temperatures at thirty thousand feet. His kidneys had failed and he barely had a heartbeat, and yet twenty-four hours later, he made a complete recovery. He was the world's first documented case of accidental human hibernation.

In 1999, near Narvik, Norway, Anna Bagenholm fell into an icy river while skiing. She spent over an hour underwater before she was recovered from her icy tomb. There seemed little hope for her recovery, but Anna was brought to the intensive care unit at Tromsø University Hospital, hooked up to a heart-lung machine, and treated by attending physician Mads Gilbert.

Anna didn't have a heartbeat or any detectable pulse; her EKG showed a flat line. By all standard definitions, she was dead. Despite her bleak prospects, the doctors kept working. Four hours after her plunge into the icy water, Anna's heart quivered and shortly thereafter began to beat normally. Anna's recovery took several months, and she has some lasting nerve damage, although no brain damage. Today she is living a normal, healthy life, working as a radiologist at the hospital that saved her life. One lasting message of her ordeal was echoed by an anesthesiologist at that hospital: "Never give up, never give up, never give up."

In October 2006, while attending a work-related barbecue on Mount Rokkō in western Japan, Mitsutaka Uchikoshi went for a brief walk during a blinding snowstorm. He accidentally slid down the side of a steep, snow-covered embankment. Mitsutaka lay undiscovered in a coma for twenty-four days. His remarkable survival was attributed to accidental human hibernation. He is alive and well today.

COOLING THERAPY

The potential for human hibernation shows great promise to hospital trauma centers around the world. Both small and large animals that are not natural hibernators have been induced to hibernate under controlled conditions. The hope is that critical patients may be cooled, which reduces the demands of the body and gives them *time* to get to a hospital. This time delay could allow bold lifesaving treatment of accident victims and many other urgent-care trauma cases, with results approaching the miraculous.

The book *Cheating Death* was published in 2009 by Dr. Sanjay Gupta, neurosurgeon and chief medical correspondent for CNN News. He presented the surprising results of cold therapy (hypothermia) for heart attack, accident, shooting, and shock victims. *The New England Journal of Medicine* reported that a large number of heart attack patients who received cooling therapy survived, while a significant percentage of victims who did not receive this treatment perished.

In 2006 at the Virginia Commonwealth University Medical Center, the survival rate of cardiac victims treated with hypothermia therapy increased by 50 percent. Obviously, a patient going home to his family is a far better outcome than coma or death.

The container and system used in hospitals for hypothermia therapy cooling cost about twenty-five thousand dollars, not a large amount of money compared with the majority of medical equipment and considering its potential to save so many lives.

At the time only a few hundred hospitals in the United States have installed these cooling units, a low number compared with the six thousand hospitals that have not added hypothermia to their heart attack treatment repertoire. Since Dr. Gupta published *Cheating Death*, more hospitals across the country have climbed aboard the hypothermia therapy train. One understandable reason for the delay is the possibility of lawsuits if the patient dies after receiving this new therapy. I know from personal experience that the fear of being sued severely restricts a doctor's confidence in trying new methods. Despite that liability, we must still forge our way ahead to such promising new procedures. It is a constant balancing act between approving a damaging treatment too soon, which directly causes someone's death, and stalling on a promising treatment, which results in needless deaths.

For years therapeutic hypothermia has been an accepted treatment for cardiac victims in Europe and to a lesser extent in Australia. Despite the large number of cardiac survivors in countries that employ hypothermia therapy, its acceptance in the United States has been delayed by conservative medical authorities.

It seems that in life-or-death situations, people's desire for heroic treatment is quite varied. Many people want no extraordinary procedures used to save their life. Others, like my mother, asked the doctors to use every treatment known to medical science to fight off her death; she intended to battle the Grim Reaper to the very end.

Nevertheless, a simple seven-degree drop in body temperature will often have an enormous positive effect on whether a cardiac arrest patient will live or die.

Think about it. *Seven degrees.*

I am not talking about expensive equipment here; I'm talking about ice.

TECHNOLOGICAL ADVANCEMENTS

Today many types of biological material are routinely frozen and stored for years and then warmed to resume functionality. These include human sperm, eggs, small embryos, and skin and blood; insects; fish; frogs; numerous seeds; and much more.

In the mid-1960s at Kobe University, Japan, Dr. Isamu Suda perfused a cat's brain with glycerol and froze it for six months. When rewarmed, the cat brain recorded an EEG not greatly different from normal.

In 2006 Kaitlyne McNamara received a new bladder, one grown from her own cells in a laboratory. This was the world's first human organ grown in a laboratory.

In 2008, for the first time in history, a heart belonging to a rat was grown in the laboratory by Dr. Doris Taylor, whose philosophy is "Give nature the tools, and get out of the way." The rat's beating heart was showcased by Dr. Anthony Atala of Wake Forest University on the *Oprah Winfrey Show* along with myriad other medical wonders to come. Can the human heart be far behind?

Stem-cell research is emerging as the most exciting and promising treatment and potential cure for all diseases known today. Many leading scientists believe that stem-cell research will extend the human life span by curing disease and greatly slowing the aging process.

In 2005 Dr. Gregory Fahy announced that his company, Twenty-First Century Medicine, had cooled a rabbit kidney down to -200°F and then warmed and implanted it back into the rabbit as the sole kidney. That rabbit's subsequent survival portends the eventual survival of us all. This is an enormous breakthrough!

Many of the world's great discoveries stem from government research and support. The military is trying to buy time for soldiers who have been critically wounded on the battlefield by artificially inducing human hibernation. With this procedure, a mortally wounded soldier with thirty minutes of life remaining could acquire several hours of time to be transferred to a hospital and prevent the ultimate sacrifice.

NASA has sent several rovers to Mars that have been searching for water and signs of life for years. Scientists now hypothesize that oceans of water once covered Mars, and scientists are on the brink of confirming that life has and does indeed exist elsewhere. This will be one of the most profound realizations humanity has ever faced.

A sensational wonder is the incredible science of nanotechnology—the world of the insanely small. This branch of medicine is so remarkable that even I, probably one of the world's most optimistic people, have trouble foreseeing the trajectory of this young science. I am glad the governments of our world are pouring billions of dollars into this research. Just one example of what may soon be possible is a tiny robot, the size of a single cell, that will be placed into an artery and travel to the damaged site in a stroke victim. Once there, it will repair all damage, including any heart damage.

FUTURE POTENTIAL OF CRYONICS

Is liquid nitrogen time travel truly possible? Will we ever be able to slow a human biological clock to within a fraction of absolute zero, hold someone there for a couple hundred years, and then return that suspended body back into a rejuvenated, thriving human being? These questions are at the soul of the cryonics quagmire.

Imagine that the human race will someday have a choice about when we are ready to give up the ghost. Yes, it will take time to perfect the cryonic suspension procedures required to resuscitate a suspended patient, but that should not keep us from climbing aboard a cryonics time machine. Almost every suspension patient has left instructions not to be resuscitated until it is medically possible to return the body to a healthful, youthful, and, some even stipulate, handsome state.

We realize we have a long wait until these dreams can be realized. But when suspended in a state-of-the-art liquid nitrogen cryonics capsule at the Cryonics Institute in Michigan or the Alcor Foundation in Arizona, the passing time will be irrelevant to the patients waiting for these miracles to materialize.

Hospitals' routinely staving off death by applying cryonic suspension is likely still decades away, but the outlook is improving. Several companies, including Florida-based Suspended Animation, Inc., are advancing toward ideal conditions for cryonic suspensions.

For almost fifty years, Saul Kent, cofounder of CSNY and now CEO of Suspended Animation, has remained a driving force in bringing the science of extended life to the public and to the world. The cryobiology conference sponsored by his company has brought many leading scientists and medical experts into cryonics. His facility offers the most advanced cryonics standby preparations, and while they are not cheap, they provide the best chance of revival. I consider him on par with Robert Ettinger as one of the most influential leaders of life extension.

Since the first cryonic suspension forty-five years ago, roughly 2.3 billion people worldwide have died. During that time about two hundred people have been placed into cryonic suspension. Even now, only about a dozen cryonics perfusions are performed each year.

The cryonics movement has gone on for twenty-five years now without my participation and has produced two state-of-the-art cryopreservation centers. There are perhaps a thousand more like me who have made all the arrangements, legal and financial, to be cryonically suspended at clinical death. I bow to everyone who will come after me, carrying the torch to a new generation. The times they are a-changing.

What might the future hold for cryonics? My hope is that by using the methods available today we can sufficiently preserve human patients so that one day technology can return them to a new life. I understand that most people will reject this option whether revival is guaranteed or not. But those few who would choose life over death should not be dismayed if some experts are not yet on our side.

The Society for Cryobiology has been hostile to cryonics since the 1960s and remains almost as hostile today. In 1965 they rejected human cryonic suspension because they could see no way to ever revive a frozen human body; at that time, not a single organ—human or animal—had ever been frozen and revived. Professor Ettinger countered them: "Of course no one today knows how a frozen patient could be resuscitated. We are not suggesting that. We are banking on future technology, and you cannot know what will be possible in the future! The future is unknown."

Throughout my cryonics experience, I have often said that we were counting on future generations to develop the necessary technology to revive frozen patients. I never imagined that I would be relying on *today's* generation!

Dr. Mark Roth, a reduced metabolism scientist at the Fred Hutchinson Cancer Research Center in Seattle, Washington, might have just struck gold. I first learned of his work in Dr. Gupta's book *Cheating Death*. Dr. Roth is using, of all things, hydrogen sulfide to reduce the body's need for oxygen. The "rotten egg" smell of hydrogen sulfide gas is instantly recognizable, and the gas can be harmful to humans at high doses. Nevertheless, Dr. Roth has found a method of creating a liquid form of hydrogen sulfide that can be injected into patients by medics on the battlefield or by EMS paramedics at an accident scene. He has discovered that when administered to a rat, the substance will induce a suspended animation–like state. The doctor's ability to take an inauspicious, potentially harmful compound like this and transform it into an agent that saves lives seems like modern-day alchemy!

His method can be practically described as a "pause switch" for death. For six hours the rat was hovering between life and death with metabolism at 10 percent of normal. When returned to an oxygenated environment, the rat made a full recovery. This procedure bought the rat six hours of time. If mortally wounded, this additional time would have allowed the rat to reach a hospital and receive lifesaving treatment.

The potential of this amazing research has caused the US Government Defense Advanced Research Projects Agency (DARPA) to fund Dr. Roth's research in suspended animation in hopes of saving the lives of soldiers wounded on the battlefield. Perfected, this science could provide hospitals with a revolutionary tool to prevent impending death. Several other researchers have also committed their resources to perfecting therapeutic human suspended animation.

In order to gain FDA approval of clinical trials, Dr. Roth had to demonstrate that 75 percent of animals recovered after losing 60 percent of their blood and being left untouched for six hours. Dr. Roth's lab accomplished this amazing feat with his pause button for death. The so-called golden hour, the time after an injury to perform lifesaving treatment, is growing by hours and days or perhaps even months. Indeed, such a pause switch for death will surely count as one of the great accomplishments of human history.

Because of his remarkable success, Dr. Roth's lab has won approval to begin human suspended animation clinical trials. The second and third phases of this research will take up to five more years to complete. The amazing reality is that reduced metabolism research on human hibernation and suspended animation is actually occurring at this very moment.

PHILOSOPHICAL RAMIFICATIONS
In the late 1960s, while president of the CSC, I commissioned a poll of random passersby at the corner of Beverly and Wilshire Boulevards in Beverly Hills, California. Although the poll was nonscientific, I wanted to gauge the reactions of Americans to cryonics. Seven CSC members spent five hours speaking with approximately four hundred people about

their familiarity with cryonics and what they might feel regarding their own cryonic suspension.

The results were tabulated—and I was stunned. Eighty percent of those polled said they had heard of cryonics, and 75 percent of them, more than two hundred, thought it was already possible to freeze and revive a human being. Of the four hundred people we queried, only eighteen (less than 5 percent) responded somewhat positively to cryonic suspension; all the rest wanted no part of extended life through cryonics or any other medical treatment. I doubt those results have changed significantly in the intervening years.

From that survey and a lifetime of anecdotal evidence, I believe children between the ages of five and seven learn that death is a routine part of life and that sooner or later everyone dies. Most simply accept death as the natural order of life.

People typically deal with death by embracing a perceived higher power. Primitive cultures had beliefs in a spirit world that ruled the forces of nature and had powers over life and death. Other civilizations embraced religious or supernatural ideas such as resurrection, reincarnation, mummification, angels, zombies, ghosts, and many others. Many such beliefs continue today.

For me the difference between the faith-based religions and science is that science is verifiable and therefore, I believe, the central author of creation. That is not to say I do not believe in God, because I do. I give all the credit and credibility of science to the power I call God. I believe that all science delivered to man over these past few centuries has been freely given by our Creator. Man cannot out-slick the Creator, by whatever name he is known. Thus I believe that science provides the gateway to new discovery. The path to future enlightenment means probing all possibilities, including what is unknown, strange, and alien.

I have learned over the past five decades since first reading *The Prospect of Immortality* that the chains of tradition are nearly impossible to break; consequently, change happens very slowly and at its own pace. Extended life via cryonics is truly only available to those rare individuals who can embrace this newly evolved possibility. Such thinkers are not conditioned to expect death at the young age of eighty when they can live as long as Methuselah. The rest of the world's billions of people will simply experience an early death and be consumed by worms or flames—which is very much their right, if not what the more-hopeful minority of us would choose. For centuries life expectancy was far lower than it is today, but medicine and technological advancements have allowed people to add decades to life. Cryonics is a natural extension of that medical and technological evolution.

There always will be reactionaries at the other end of consciousness who distrust the evolving knowledge of the human mind. However, we should not dampen our optimism about the great benefits that future discoveries can deliver.

Two hundred years ago, flying among the clouds would have been miraculous, an astonishing gift of the gods. Now it is ordinary, even boring. With each new invention and discovery, our perceptions shift. If you could talk to a caveman today, do you think he would be convinced that airplanes, skydiving parachutes, and submarines are now commonplace?

For now there are questions to consider: Why should we hope that a future generation will revive frozen human beings of our time? What has the cryonics movement accomplished or discovered over these past fifty years? How might those accomplishments support the enormous effort to greatly extend the human life span?

*   *   *

To witness your own proof of principle and perhaps re-create some of the magic I felt when I first observed the sea monkeys, I propose that you supercool some ordinary houseflies in your home refrigerator for a few days and then bring them back to life.

First catch a few healthy flies. I usually just place something like a banana peel on an outside table, and while the flies are busy chomping away, I trap them with a clear glass. This method works well for me, although I needed some practice and had to move fast.

When I've captured a half dozen, I place them in a covered clear glass and put them in the refrigerator. Within a few minutes they appear dead, lying on their backs, feet straight up. They have, by all appearances, gone to the happy buzzing grounds. What is going on here? Are these flies dead? Are they alive even though they appear to be dead? The flies are in a "pause mode," what Dr. Sanjay Gupta suggests would be the greatest medical discovery in the history of medicine if it can be applied to humans.

Sometime within the next three days, assemble an audience to witness your amazing live-giving powers. Take the glass out of the refrigerator, head outside, and drop the flies onto your palm. After about three minutes, the warmth of your palm will reinvigorate the flies; as if by magic, they will suddenly stand up, shake a little, and shortly thereafter fly off. While this is a cute parlor trick, it does illustrate in a small way the slowing down of biological life.

I suggest searching for *cryonics* on the Internet and learning more about its current status from enlightening presentations by the Cryonics Institute and Alcor Foundation on their websites. You might be impressed to learn about the number and caliber of the scientists and professionals who have joined this young science.

Cryonics information and discussions are easily found. Two popular online forums are Cryonet and The Cold Filter. I also suggest reading *Cheating Death*, mentioned earlier, and *Engines of Creation* by Eric Drexler, a cryonics suspension member. His book portrays the revolution of new medicine including cryonics, stem cell research, and cloning.

We must use our own imagination to decide whether we want to participate in extending our lives into the near and distant future. There is a suicide somewhere in the world every twenty seconds—a statistic proving that life is often very tenuous, depending on a person's circumstances.

George Sanders was a favorite silver screen idol of mine during the 1960s; his charming manner coupled with good looks and a rich voice gifted him with an Academy Award, fame, fortune, and talent—everything I thought a reasonable person would prize.

In 1971, just prior to committing suicide, George Sanders wrote this note:

Dear friends, I am leaving this world because I am bored. I have lived long enough. I am leaving you, with all your worries, in this sweet cesspool of life. Good luck!

The prospect of cryonics, if successful, would challenge our belief systems and traditions. It would change the way we view and deal with death. Our world is inhabited by billions of dissimilar people who tend to not recognize or embrace change—especially change that radically transforms life as we have lived it for eons.

I once heard a story about President Theodore Roosevelt's reaction when his secretary of state told him that the Wright brothers had just achieved the first human flight at Kitty Hawk. While he was stunned and amazed, he commented that he could see no practical application for it!

If that story was retold correctly, then for me it exemplifies what I call "looking versus seeing." Even this great president could not see the potential for human flight to change the world. In 1967, when the first heart transplant took place, a majority of people were shocked and even appalled. Yet today heart transplants are a commonly practiced and accepted form of life extension.

Today only a handful of people *look* at cryonics and the science of reduced metabolism and *see* its world-changing potential. I saw its potential. I imagined a world where dying was simply an option. It's what drove me to act with passion and persistence, sacrificing everything I had for an idea that would usher the evolution of man to superman.

I leave you now by reiterating the assessment of CNN chief medical correspondent Dr. Sanjay Gupta of suspended animation: "This could be the biggest medical breakthrough ever—a way to stop death in its tracks."

The day we humans are able to defeat death may soon be at hand. Think about it!

Status & Prospects
R. C. W. Ettinger[*]

BOB NELSON'S STORY SPEAKS FOR ITSELF. No need to gild the lily, so I'll just add a few notes from my perspective.

Life is stranger than art, but not as neat. Good guys usually have a few warts, and bad guys are sometimes kind to their dogs. Smart people can do dumb things, and banal people occasionally show common sense. But both brilliance and common sense will have a struggle against habits ingrained over thousands of generations.

How to cut the chains of tradition? It can be done in minutes, acetylene torch style, by the white-hot passion of a Bob Nelson, but this is rare indeed. It can also be done file-style, sawing away patiently. Or if we change the metaphor to that of a dungeon prisoner, he might dig his way out with a spoon, working year after year—in other words, you can slowly build your information and determination.

In 1962 I published the first version of *The Prospect of Immortality;* the first commercial edition was published in 1964. Since then, no one has managed to live forever.

In 1972 the first edition of my *Man into Superman* was published. Since then, no one has leaped any tall buildings.

Still, there has been progress. It has been much less rapid than I originally hoped, and the cryonics movement remains very small, with only around a thousand people actively involved and only around 170 patients in frozen storage, or cryostasis, as of the beginning of 2008. Even the broader "immortalist" movement remains small; few acknowledge, even to themselves, that the total elimination of death might not be a bad thing and that the possibility should be investigated.

But the still broader "life extension" movement is going great guns, with many millions of people trying to improve their lifestyles and buying

---

[*] Ettinger wrote this epilogue in 2008 before he died and was suspended.

dietary supplements touted as life-extending. Billions of dollars are being spent on the development of nanotechnology, or molecular engineering, the potential of which includes submicroscopic robots to maintain and repair the human body from the inside. Every year, almost every day, advances in science and technology make our thesis more credible.

There are also solid indications of an acceleration of progress, one example being that the Cryonics Institute, started in 1976, froze its first patient (my mother) in 1977 but has received more than half of its current eighty-five patients in the past five years. Membership has more than tripled in the last seven years. The wind is at our backs, even if it is still just a light breeze.

Perhaps I should not have been surprised at the slow growth. After all, one could regard the cryonics/immortalist movement as the most radical revolution in human history, with a perceivable threat to many of the habits and institutions that people hold dear. Perhaps the real surprise is that it has taken root and grown, and no one has even been lynched. (Cryonics has been effectively outlawed in a few places, such as France and the Canadian province of British Columbia, but in the United States the opposition has been mostly just a few grumbles. And there are countries, such as Australia, where interest per capita is higher than in the United States.)

As for interest in trans-humanity—forget it, for now. Oh, there is plenty of intellectual interest or fantasizing, and there has been for a long time. Science fiction is around a hundred years old as a popular genre, and many of the biggest movie hits of recent decades have been of this sort. Science fiction is now a *major* part of the entertainment scene. But fictional supermen have very rarely shown any genuine superiority worth mentioning, for the simple reason that readers would not relate to them and writing about them would be too difficult, if possible at all.

In fact, very few people want radical change of any kind. They want their idealized future to be just like the present, except gold-plated or chocolate-covered. Or we could say they want the present without warts—nothing much different except more money and less suffering, along with continued life. And it's hard to quarrel with that.

The future is almost certain to be rowdier than we would like, and the surprises will not all be pleasant. Some of the heavy thinkers believe that within the next fifty years, or even sooner, accelerating scientific advances will bring the "spike" or "singularity"—a sudden surge of change (including intelligent machines and self-reproducing factories) that will compress centuries of change into years. That is downright frightening. But playing ostrich won't help, and if there is much to worry about, there is probably more to hope for.

WHAT KIND OF PEOPLE ARE INVOLVED IN CRYONICS?

It is mildly interesting to glance at the record for clues as to what kind of people are attracted to—or repelled by—the concepts of cryonics and immortalism, or life extension. There are some surprises.

Early on, some of the professional chatterers warned that the cryonics "scam" would seduce countless of the desperate aged to throw their money at the body-freezers. That never happened, and would not have happened even if we had been ambulance chasers and even if we were in it for the money, which is verifiably not the case.

Old people naturally dominate our patient rolls, but the aged are not our best potential recruits by any means. They seldom have any strong fear of death or any strong will to live, or much ability to think outside the box or deviate from the ordinary. Typically, all they want is surcease or respite. They descend passively into oblivion.

Their children, or in some cases their spouses, may take a different view. The majority of members of the cryonics organizations are men, but the majority of patients are women. They are the mothers and wives who were held especially dear, and given their chance. Next most frequent patients are fathers and husbands.

What about occupation?

Cryonicists cover a broad spectrum, with clearly a concentration of the better educated. For example, we like to say that "doctors choose cryonics, nine to one."

That doesn't mean 90 percent of physicians are in cryonics. The absolute numbers are small in every segment of the population. But we do have about nine times as many physicians in cryonics as you would expect on the basis of population. In other words, a doctor is about nine times as likely to be involved in cryonics as a person chosen at random from the population. If we look at PhDs, the numbers are even more striking.

Computer professionals are even more highly overrepresented, and we have a theory about that. Computer people not only depend on logic on a day-to-day basis but are also accustomed to seeing rapid advances in what is possible.

One cannot say the same thing about any other profession. Lawyers use logic, but the law changes very slowly, and judges and juries may disregard logic. Medicine involves logic, but a lot of it is guesswork, and clinical proof of effectiveness and FDA approval come very slowly. Engineers use logic, but much of what they do requires lots of capital, and again change is slow. The computer field is unique in its total reliance on logic and the ease and rapidity of improvements—and that, we think, makes computer people unusually open to our thesis.

Personality? There hasn't been any scientific survey, but we do know for example that Libertarians are overrepresented in cryonics. The main characteristic of Libertarians is independence and love of freedom, with distrust of authority. Many of them are entrepreneurs, self-employed. I don't endorse the Libertarian political party, but they are interesting people and less likely than most to be chained to old habits.

The bottom line of course is that the "typical" cryonicist profile really doesn't matter. The one thing that matters is whether you and your family will survive and thrive. At present, a majority [of people] are skeptical of cryonics—so will you let that majority vote you into the grave?

HEROES AND ZEROES

Many people are people-people, responding better to human-interest stories than to dry logic. So let me relate a few of our stories, or at least their brief versions. The "zeroes" are of two sorts: those who are moldering and those who look like long shots but still have a chance. The "heroes" are also of two sorts: those who tried and failed and those who tried and have a chance. I won't specify in advance which is which.

Walt Disney

According to the gossip, Walt had heard about cryonics and expressed his desire to be frozen at death. According to the persistent rumor, he actually was frozen, privately, and is hidden away somewhere. My tentative conclusion is that he did express such a wish but took no concrete steps to assure it, and when he died, he lost a lot of influence. His family thought his wishes were less important than their business, and they buried him—a grave mistake from his point of view, and ours. At any rate, there is a grave in a California cemetery with a Walt Disney marker on it.

So Mickey Mouse is immortal, in his fashion, but his daddy is probably just dead.

Andrea Foote

Dr. Foote was a psychologist on the faculty of the University of Michigan and served on the board of directors of the Cryonics Institute for many years. When she was dying of cancer, arrangements were made to keep her at home under hospice care, with family members (who cooperated with her wishes) in attendance and Cryonics Institute equipment in place. We were prepared; she was promptly perfused and frozen and is now at the Cryonics Institute facility in Clinton Township, Michigan, northeast of Detroit. She left CI a bequest of more than one hundred thousand dollars.

Note: No director or officer of the Cryonics Institute is paid a penny or derives any financial benefit from its operations. There are no stockholders. It is a nonprofit organization run by the members for the benefit of the patients. CI received the bulk of Professor Ettinger's estate after his clinical death and he was frozen.

We have nothing against capitalism and expect and hope that the likes of General Electric, Frigidaire, etc., may eventually enter the field. But we need to squelch the suspicion that CI or its directors are in it for the money. We are in it for something more valuable—to save our lives and those of the people we love.

Richard Jones

Professional name Dick Clair, he was a TV writer and producer, especially for *The Carol Burnett Show*. He was signed up at various times with three different cryonics organizations, the last being Alcor, where he is currently safely stored. He left his estate to Alcor, but the inevitable litigation by heirs resulted in a split settlement. Alcor did, however, receive a substantial bequest, I think over a million dollars. This was Alcor's chief asset for years. Definitely a hero.

Stanley Kubrick

The famous director of *Dr. Strangelove, 2001: A Space Odyssey*, and many other films saw me on one of the TV shows—I think it was *Tonight* with Johnny Carson—bought dozens of copies of my book *The Prospect of Immortality*, and invited me to New York to meet some of his rich friends. Unfortunately, he also invited a scientist/businessman named Ben Schloss, who apparently conned him out of some money and thereby soured his interest.

Peter Sellers

The actor (*Pink Panther, Being There, Dr. Strangelove*, etc.) had a flash of interest and wrote me a warm letter, but he had a short attention span and of course many other interests competing for his attention. He ended in a grave or crematory, I don't know which.

Don Laughlin

Possibly the flashiest of current living cryonics members is the man with a city named for him—Laughlin, Nevada, a kind of junior Las Vegas centered around his casino resort. Laughlin is a billionaire, or half anyway, so who says rich people can't be smart? And don't say he's a gambler, because his habits couldn't be more different from those of his customers. He only places bets when the odds are in his favor. Does that tell you something?

K. Eric Drexler

Dr. Drexler is a shaker and mover in the massive scientific drive loosely called nanotechnology, or molecular engineering. Very roughly speaking, this means building things by moving individual atoms, one at a time. Drexler's first book, *Engines of Creation,* was published about the same time, 1986, that two IBM scientists built the first scanning tunneling microscope, which could "see" and even manipulate individual atoms. Drexler foresees computer-driven machines (assemblers), which will be able to build almost anything—including copies of themselves!—out of almost any raw material, such as air, water, or dirt, using any available energy, such as sunlight.

Such devices already exist in nature of course. They are called plants. But those prospectively designed and built by humans will be much more versatile. Remember the movie *Fantastic Voyage* with Raquel Welch, where a submarine carrying doctors was miniaturized and injected into the bloodstream of a patient to carry out repairs? That was silly—wasn't it? Yes, but it isn't silly to envision ultraminiaturized robots—nanobots—that could do the same thing. They could also repair the damage done by freezing a cryonics patient.

Yes, one of our greatest heroes, Dr. Drexler is a cryonicist.

Richard Feynman

Professor Feynman won a Nobel prize in physics for contributions to quantum theory, the forefront of physics. In 1958 he gave a lecture, "Plenty of Room at the Bottom," explaining his opinion that no known law prevented our learning how to manipulate atoms individually, with the implication that we could design and build—and repair!—physical systems of any complexity (such as you). This came to the attention of a young student, K. Eric Drexler, who proceeded to do something about it, as already noted.

Dr. Feynman saw the promised land, however dimly; but, like Moses, he didn't get there. Perhaps due to cultural inertia, he did nothing about cryonics and died a few years ago. A partial hero.

VITRIFICATION PROGRESS

A great many people who ought to know better—including not only physicians but even professional cryobiologists, "experts" in low temperature biology—have said that freezing ruptures cells because water expands when it freezes, and the idea of repairing all the billions of ruptured cells in a human body is preposterous.

The fact is, first, that animal cell walls are elastic, and the expansion of water when it freezes is only about 10 percent, which could mostly be accommodated. More importantly, however, it just isn't true that cells burst when a large specimen (such as a person) is frozen slowly (the only possible kind of freezing for large specimens, barring methods involving high pressure). Instead water is *withdrawn* from the cells and freezes in the intercellular spaces, so the cells, far from bursting, actually shrink.

That doesn't mean freezing is harmless. There can still be mechanical damage by ice crystals tearing cell walls, for example. There will also be chemical damage, because when water is withdrawn from cells, the remaining solution becomes hypertonic, with solutes too concentrated, and proteins may become denatured, etc.

But we mustn't overdo the pessimism. Despite the difficulties, a great many biological specimens have in fact been completely frozen, stored at liquid nitrogen temperature, and then revived. These include not only microscopic forms of life, and a few insects, but also a few adult mammalian organs, such as the rat ovary and rat parathyroid. There have also been many partial successes, such as recovery of hamsters to normal behavior after half the water in their brains had been changed to ice. Microscopic and other studies show that our procedures greatly reduce the damage that would otherwise occur. (There is much more detail on the CI website: www.cryonics.org.)

But even though freezing leaves realistic hope, it would still be better if we could avoid ice formation. And there is indeed such a thing as solidification by cold without ice formation. It is called vitrification, which means formation of a glass-like condition.

Glasses, and similar substances such as tars, which are liquid when hot, can cool and become apparently solid, yet not form the crystals typical of solids. Instead they retain the ability to flow, very slowly. Over periods of many years, glass windowpanes may observably settle, becoming slightly thicker at the bottom.

Certain water solutions can also vitrify under appropriate conditions. When Dr. Yuri Pichugin was director of research at the Cryonics Institute, he developed new and improved vitrification solutions and procedures, which are undergoing continued and extended tests. We do not foresee that, anytime soon, procedures will be so highly perfected that a healthy person could be vitrified and immediately revived—let alone someone who has died of old age or disease or trauma, or someone who suffered a long delay between death and cryopreservation. But hope continues, and grows.

The bottom line is the same. For the first time in human history, there is a realistic chance of rescue of so-called "dead" people. How good that chance may be, and how much you value it, are questions for you to decide.

ACKNOWLEDGMENTS

Professor Robert Ettinger: My mentor and the father of the cryonics generation.

Frank Enderle: The first cemetery director to allow cryonic suspension patients to be interred on cemetery grounds.

Saul Kent: A founder of the very first cryonics organization, the Cryonics Society of New York, and president of Florida-based Suspended Animation. He's a giant in the world of cryonics.

Curtis Henderson: The first president of the Cryonics Society of New York.

Ben Best: Until recently, president of the Michigan-based Cryonics Institute, now maintaining more than 120 frozen patients.

Andy Zawacki: Caretaker of the CI suspension facility—he does it all!

Mike Perry: One of my favorite people in the world of cryonics. A cryonics historian for more than thirty years, he's legendary for tenaciously digging to always find the truth. His tireless pursuit of the truth and endless fact-checking of the manuscript were instrumental in making this memoir as accurate as humanly possible.

York Porter: Executive editor of the *Long Life* cryonics newsletter, which covers every aspect of what is going on in the world of cryonics.

John Bull: Former editor of the *Long Life* newsletter. He's a gentleman and unsurpassed in his ability to get the written word to the public.

Jim Yount: Chairman of the San Francisco–based cryonics group of millionaires who have made all legal and financial arrangements to be suspended—and to take their money with them.

Alcor Life Extension Foundation: Alcor is one of two facilities currently accepting cryonics patients in the United States. This was made possible by the death of cryonics member Dick Jones, who left several million dollars to the cryonics movement for his own suspension. The brilliant work of Fred and Linda Chamberlain in bringing this cryonics facility into existence is comparable, in my opinion, to Neil Armstrong being first man on the moon. And whenever the first man is revived, I believe Alcor will be viewed as an even greater accomplishment.

Cryonics Institute: Robert Ettinger was the champion of bringing the Cryonics Institute into existence. This futuristic marvel, in my view, is a first-class cryonics suspension facility that has faced and resolved all the legal, financial, and engineering issues that are unique to this futuristic choice of embracing greatly extended life. Alcor and Cryonics Institute presently have 118 suspensions making a total of 236 human patients. There are, on average, 180 suicides somewhere in the world every hour, every day. That translates into every twenty-four hours, a total of 4,320 human beings choose death over life. So it seems that life itself, let alone extended life, is not for everyone!

My daughter Susan has been my right arm and my strongest supporter of life extension; she was there befriending little Genevieve's suspension and is here at my side this very moment—I thank you from the bottom of my heart, my beautiful daughter. My daughter Lori has been a staunch supporter of my cryonics activities and has been a pioneering spirit in support of her dad's adventures into extended life.

My two youngest daughters—Christine, now twenty-two, and Natalie, just weeks away from turning eighteen—are products of growing up in a world that today looks at extended life as a good thing and simply a part of our Creator's loving revelations to our ever-changing world.

My son John was my first child; he passed away from heart disease. You are dearly missed, my son.

Clyde, Elaine, and Valerie Smith are my precious fans and most dearly loved.

The shining star of my return to cryonics after a twenty-five-year absence goes to my wife, Moeurth. She reignited the trembling happiness of life.

My coauthor Kenneth Bly would like to thank his mother, Connie Mayo, and his nephew, Ryan Hall, for putting up with several years when all he could talk about was cryonics. His mother often told him to "take a break from all this dead people stuff and go out and get laid." She passed away before the book was finished, God bless her soul. Also, he acknowledges Nancy Groesbeck for her loving support through his mother's illness and the writing of this book.

My coauthor Sally Magaña wishes to thank her husband, Quetzalcoatl Magaña, for his unparalleled clarity and keen insights.

Last but far from least is a powerful left arm, the daughter of Sandra Stanley, my coauthor on *We Froze the First Man*: Jonna Jetson Coleman. Her skill in public relations and management is always an enormous aid in my journey of getting the world to not only look at the cryonics thesis of life extension but to *actually see it!* Jonna has blossomed into a new generation leader in recognizing that the Creator himself is the enlightener of evolutionary revelations that allow humanity to evolve into beings of an almost heavenly spiritual realm.

ABOUT THE AUTHORS

Bob Nelson is the author of *We Froze the First Man* and was president of the Cryonics Society of California. In 1967 he froze the first man. He has made appearances with Regis Philbin and Phil Donahue and on NPR's *This American Life*. His story is being adapted into a major motion picture featuring a star-studded cast. He lives in Oceanside, California.

Kenneth Bly worked with Bob Nelson at his electronics repair center from 1995 to 2003, when Bob retired. He spent several years researching Bob's role in cryonics and worked closely with Bob to write the basic manuscript. He currently works from his home in Oceanside, California.

Sally Magaña received her PhD in chemical engineering. Previously, she coauthored a novel, *Lost Hope,* about the Hope Diamond with her husband, Quetzalcoatl Magaña.

www.facebook.com/Freezing.People.Is.Not.Easy